MW01075376

VOICES OF
Recovery

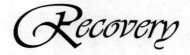

A DAILY READER
SECOND EDITION

ISBN 978-1-889681-42-9
Library of Congress Control Number: 2021949879

Overeaters Anonymous, Inc.
World Service Office
6075 Zenith Court NE
Rio Rancho, NM 87144-6424 USA
Mail Address: P.O. Box 44727
Rio Rancho, NM 87174-4727 USA
1-505-891-2664
info@oa.org
www.oa.org

VOICES OF

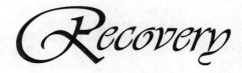
Recovery

A DAILY READER
SECOND EDITION

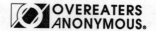
OVEREATERS ANONYMOUS.

Foreword

*O*ver a period of three years, a worldwide call went out to the members of the OA Fellowship asking them to submit quotations from OA literature that have helped them in working the program and to reflect on how those words continue to inspire them in their recovery.

Over eight hundred personal expressions of experience, strength, and hope were received, and 366 were chosen by fellow OA members for inclusion in this daily reader. The quotations came from such Conference- and Board-approved literature as *The Twelve Steps and Twelve Traditions of Overeaters Anonymous, For Today, Abstinence, The Tools of Recovery,* and *Beyond Our Wildest Dreams.*

These voices of recovery do not represent OA as a whole; they are written as a loving service by OA members for OA members.

Foreword to the Second Edition

*I*n preparing this second edition, all of the quotations used as inspiration for the original passages submitted by members of the Fellowship were reviewed and edited to bring them into alignment with OA's currently available literature. In most cases, the quotations required only editing of punctuation, updating of a citation to a new edition, or editing of a few words. Where the quoted piece of literature had been discontinued or the quotation had been entirely eliminated in the newer version of the literature, new quotations that would still honor the spirit of the original writing were painstakingly sought. The replacement quotations were chosen from newer Conference- and Board-approved literature, such as the second edition of *The Twelve Steps and Twelve Traditions of Overeaters Anonymous,* the third edition of *Overeaters Anonymous,* the second edition of *Abstinence, Taste of Lifeline,* and some of the more recently approved pamphlets.

In only a couple of cases, it was thought to be essential to make minor word changes to the original writing in order to both keep its message and bring it into alignment with current literature and policy.

It was always the intention during the review for this second edition of *Voices of Recovery* to honor the writings chosen for the first edition that have become so much a part of so many OA members' recovery.

Table of *Contents*

JAN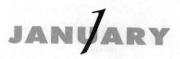UARY

> *"We admitted we were powerless over food—that our lives had become unmanageable."*
>
> —Step One

When I first came to OA, I had already lost ninety pounds, but I was struggling and knew I needed help. As soon as I walked through the door to my first meeting, I knew I was in the right place. I thought I had taken Step One that first night—certainly I was powerless over food or I wouldn't be here.

I continued to eat the same way I had been eating. I ate all foods but limited the quantities of my favorites. I didn't have any binge foods—no, not me. Of course, I still struggled, even though I was working the Steps. I started eating more at meals. As long as it was part of a meal, I was still abstinent, right? I only ate three meals a day.

Eventually, my Higher Power got a message through my food fog. He made me realize that I was playing with fire, still controlling my food. I had not taken Step One.

Amazingly, when I gave up my binge foods, abstinence became easy. The compulsion was lifted. Miracles happen when we work the Steps honestly!

For today, I will be honest about my binge foods.

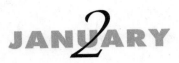
"Recovery is a journey, and the Twelve Step program is the road we travel together in OA."

—*The Twelve Steps and Twelve Traditions of Overeaters Anonymous*, 2nd ed., p. 108

My old way of thinking was that I was either an utter failure as a human being, or I was a saint. I saw myself as an utter failure; my attempts at controlling my weight and my eating only strengthened my view of myself. I dreamt of a glorious change in me: a totally compassionate, intelligent, and, of course, thin person. The trouble was that there was no road between me, the miserable failure, and me, the thin saint. So I retreated to eating and daydreaming. I used to envision a sudden flip into a different me—as if by magic I would be transformed. But OA has taught me that recovery requires patient and persistent commitment to a glorious, but hard, journey. OA has shown me the long road that leads away from failure. OA has taught me how to acknowledge my shortcomings and how, by working the Steps to change, I can drop the self-hate and humbly rely on my Higher Power. I am journeying to recovery with OA's Twelve Steps.

JAN*3*ARY

"True comfort is to be found in the balance and sanity of abstinence. So deep and pure is this comfort that it is well worth whatever trouble or pain I might have to pass through to attain it."

—For Today, p. 253

When I became newly abstinent, I went through a difficult time experiencing the pain that had been buried under food and fat. I felt it mostly at night. Up came all the aches of the past: terrors, regrets, and deep, deep sadness. I exorcised those ghosts with the help of my OA friends and the Twelve Steps. I used the Tools of telephone and writing a lot. The support I received was incredible. I'm so grateful!

Now true comfort for me is waking up with that clean, happy feeling, knowing I was abstinent the day before. True comfort is:

Hearing the birds sing

Breathing the sweet breath of life

Thrilling to the beauty of nature

Loving this moment

Loving the people I'm with

Being grateful all the time.

So deep and pure and satisfying is abstinence, I wouldn't trade it for anything.

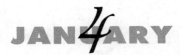

JANUARY 4

"God grant me the serenity to accept ..."
—Serenity Prayer

Am I able to accept the vicissitudes of life, the craziness, the alternating surprises and disappointments? Is it possible to accept and allow every moment of every day to be exactly as it is? Can I allow every person I meet to be exactly as he or she is at that moment?

With the help of my loving Higher Power who accepts and allows me to be exactly as I am at this moment, I can. With my dawning acceptance, I feel a peace and serenity beyond understanding.

Serenity is knowing and accepting that God is in charge.

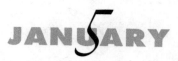
"Our common welfare should come first; personal recovery depends upon OA unity."

—Tradition One

There are at least three factions of OA. One emphasizes a strict, disciplined food plan. Another professes working the Steps and allowing God to remove the food problem. A third group falls somewhere in between. I know OA members in all three groups who have great recovery. What is the right way? What is the OA way? What is the message we are supposed to carry?

The only message I can carry is my own recovery. I do not need to have everyone recover "my way." You need the freedom to recover "your way." The only thing we need to have in common about our recovery lies within the Twelve Steps and Twelve Traditions. We cannot legislate recovery; we cannot even accurately define recovery, but we recognize it when we see someone living it.[1] Let us rejoice when we see fellow sufferers recovering in Overeaters Anonymous, thankful they have found their way. Let us be willing to try a different approach if our way is not working. Let's be open-minded and nonjudgmental. The program is broad enough for all of us to do whatever is necessary.

---

[1] Overeaters Anonymous accepts the following definitions: Abstinence is the action of refraining from compulsive eating and compulsive food behaviors while working towards or maintaining a healthy body weight. Spiritual, emotional, and physical recovery is the result of living and working the Overeaters Anonymous Twelve Step program on a daily basis. (Business Conference Policy Manual, 1988b [amended 2002, 2009, 2011, 2019, and 2021])

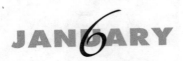

JANUARY 6

"'I can't; God can; I think I'll let God!'"

— *The Twelve Steps and Twelve Traditions of Overeaters Anonymous*, 2nd ed., p. 17

Before I came to OA, God showed me that I hurt my relationship with him when I ate sweets. I was a glutton, and I couldn't eat junk food in moderation. I vowed that I would never eat these harmful substances again. Of course, I couldn't stick to my vow! I made the vow for the right reasons, knowing by then that my weight wasn't the main issue, but I was trying to keep the vow through my own strength. Thank God for OA, which brought the reality of Steps One, Two, and Three into my life. I now trust God to do for me what I have never been able to do for myself. I am powerless over food and the rest of my life. By God's grace, I am able to stay abstinent and live in his will "one day at a time"!

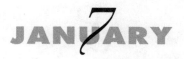

JANUARY 7

"Accept that a bite or two will not make a bad situation better."
—Think First…

My sponsor has a wonderful way of reminding me what that phrase means. When I tell her that I can't go on, she says, "If I thought that food was going to fix your husband (kid, job, etc.), I would tell you to eat. It won't."

That brings it into focus. No food exists that will make my job situation more pleasant, cure loneliness or fatigue, heal a broken relationship, or cure an illness. Eating will not fix it!

When I know this above all else, I can look at my options. The cure or solution may manifest itself when I take it to my Higher Power. Spending quiet time and listening for an answer has solved more dilemmas and cured more ills than any amount of food. Making a phone call instead of opening the refrigerator helps me find a way to handle the situation. Reading OA-approved literature, going to a meeting, or going for a walk are the things that can help me find the path I need to take.

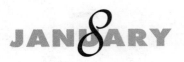

JANUARY 8

"Weaving the Fabric of Our Lives."
    —*Beyond Our Wildest Dreams*, p. 175

"Weaving the Fabric of Our Lives," chapter thirteen of *Beyond Our Wildest Dreams*, has provided me with a fresh image of the OA program and my personal recovery journey. This image reinforces for me the importance of making OA an integral part of my life. By using the Steps to guide my behavior, the Traditions to guide our groups, and the Concepts of Service to guide our service bodies, I can weave a beautiful recovery tapestry and increase my chances of staying in recovery. The image of my Higher Power lovingly guiding the weaving of my recovery tapestry—spiritual, emotional, and physical—adds to my peace and serenity. As long as I use the Tools: meetings, telephone, a plan of eating, sponsorship, writing, literature, action plan, anonymity, and service, my recovery tapestry will not unravel, and I will continue to move forward in my recovery.

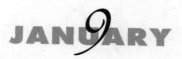
JANUARY 9

"This willingness to act on faith, then, was the key to Step Two."
—*The Twelve Steps and Twelve Traditions of Overeaters Anonymous*, 2nd ed., p. 15

Acting on faith means standing without my defenses to protect me and assuming that my Higher Power will do the right thing for me and will give me what I need, if not what I want. Acting on faith means believing my Higher Power will always listen and encourage me when I am in a situation in which I have to take risks. My Higher Power will walk with me through the scary situations and will be with me to the end when the trials are over. That's acting on faith.

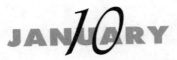

"As we become aware of what our healthy eating guidelines should be, we ask God for the willingness and the ability to live within them each day. We ask and we receive, first the willingness, and then the ability. We can count on this without fail."

—The Twelve Steps and Twelve Traditions of Overeaters Anonymous, 2nd ed., p. 21

At a time in my recovery when I could not stay abstinent, the words "without fail" offered me comfort and hope. When I could do nothing else, I could pray on my knees every day, no matter what, for the willingness and ability to be abstinent. The miracle is that the willingness came and then the ability. I continue to ask God for the willingness and ability to be abstinent daily, and it continues to work. I believe that just as God grants me the willingness and ability to be abstinent, he helps me overcome my character defects. If I pray for the willingness and ability to do God's will, I will receive the willingness and then the ability. Thank you, God!

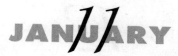

JANUARY 11

> "Step Eleven encourages us to practice *prayer*, to continue talking to our Higher Power daily, even when it seems like a senseless exercise."
>
> —*The Twelve Steps and Twelve Traditions of Overeaters Anonymous*, 2nd ed., p. 76

My first attempts at practicing prayer were a self-pitying review of my failings, or reviewing arguments for the existence of God, or crying to a God—whose existence I doubted—that I would not go to bed until he/it promised me I would be abstinent tomorrow. All these methods failed me. Because prayer appeared not to work, it was hard to keep up any consistent practice. But over the years of trial and error, repeatedly trying and failing to pray regularly, I have learned how I need to pray.

I thank God for my abstinence and my recovery. I ask for help with my abstinence in the day ahead. I offer my service. I acknowledge the previous day's failings and ask to be shown how to do better. I offer the day ahead to the service of God. I pray for friends in and out of OA. From the time I started this simple daily routine, my recovery stopped plodding forward— it sprang forward.

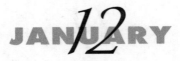

"Each morning brings a new surrender, a new admission of my powerlessness and a new commitment to abstinence through steps one, two and three. It is a quiet time, a new beginning, a new day."

—*Lifeline Sampler*, p. 69

How am I going to spend today? Will I waste it by looking at my past mistakes, or by daydreaming about what the future may hold? Living in today is often difficult. Once I let go of yesterday and tomorrow, I can live today to its fullest. Planning and dreaming will not change what my Higher Power has in store for me tomorrow, so I will turn that over and rest in the knowledge that I will be taken care of. This frees me to accept the gift of the present. It is what I do today that really matters. I can only be happy by spending today gratefully accepting who I am, what I have, and what I can do in this moment to better myself. Today will eventually become tomorrow, without my worrying or interfering with my Higher Power's plans. Let me live as if tomorrow is just another word in the dictionary. Let me live in today.

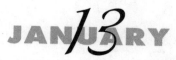

"We are neither above nor below the rest of the human race; we are a part of it."

—*The Twelve Steps and Twelve Traditions of Overeaters Anonymous*, 2nd ed., p. 41

As I finish my Fifth Step, I feel relieved and excited. I know my Higher Power has been with me all the way, prodding and leading me. I had always felt apart from the human race. I felt I had to be better than everyone else or I was no good at all. I acted out this feeling by being a "know-it-all."

As I reflected on my Fourth Step inventory, I began to realize that I was no different from any of my fellows in OA. I had heard many of these things in meetings. Why did I think I was different?

My Fifth Step process opened my eyes, and I began to see the reality of my life. I was one of many, reaching out to others and to my Higher Power, trying to get healthy.

As I talked with my sponsor, I felt humbled, accepted, and loved. I was finally part of the human race: no better and no worse than the next person. What an incredible program! Thank you, OA, my fellows, and my Higher Power.

JAN*14*ARY

"Perhaps we didn't believe that our compulsive eating was a spiritual problem, or we felt that God was concerned only with more important matters and expected us to control such a simple thing as our eating."

—*The Twelve Steps and Twelve Traditions of Overeaters Anonymous*, 2nd ed., p. 14

I remember sitting down to my first abstinent meal, which was half of what I usually ate. I thought this amount of food would never satisfy me. But I wanted to follow directions, so I ate only what was in front of me. When I spoke to my sponsor later that evening, I told her how I had felt. She suggested that at my next meal I ask God to make it enough. I really didn't believe that God could or would help me with my food, but I took her suggestion on blind faith, and it worked! I no longer use food to fill the empty places inside me; God fills me instead.

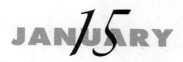
"In OA, we have discovered that humility is simply an awareness of who we really are today and a willingness to become all that we can be."

—*The Twelve Steps and Twelve Traditions of Overeaters Anonymous*, 2nd ed., p. 52

OA has given me a newfound freedom, the freedom that comes as a result of practicing unconditional love and acceptance of the person I am today.

In my Fourth and Fifth Steps, I realized what character traits and behaviors had outlived their usefulness to my life. I saw that my old ways of reaching out to the world kept me from reaching my full potential. In Step Six, I became willing to let go of whatever stood in the way of my being present to life.

I am powerless over fixing myself, but I am not helpless. I can pray for the willingness to be willing to surrender and allow the natural progression of change to unfold in God's time. I can even enjoy myself in the process.

OA has given me back my power. Today I choose to practice unconditional self-acceptance while I relish the mystery of change.

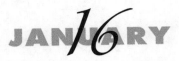
"Those of us who live this program don't simply carry the message; we are the message. Each day that we live well, we are well, and we embody the joy of recovery."

— *The Twelve Steps and Twelve Traditions of Overeaters Anonymous*, 2nd ed., pp. 86–87

When I first walked into the rooms of Overeaters Anonymous, I was like the candle whose light is flickering and close to going out. I was sick in mind, body, and spirit; I was hopeless.

Many OA members describe OA as the last house on the block. I do not know if that is true since I do not know where the block begins or ends. I do know that what I found in OA can be found only in the heart and mind of another recovering compulsive overeater. The flickering light that I came in with became stronger, and the hopelessness turned into hopefulness.

I can be a living example or a dying example of how the program works. My courage to recover and my experiences in OA serve as an example to those who know me. I represent and carry the message of hope.

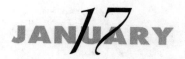

"Perseverance brings us the reward of continuing, permanent recovery."

—*The Twelve Steps and Twelve Traditions of Overeaters Anonymous*, 2nd ed., p. 86

Before I entered recovery, perseverance meant struggling through your problems and winding up eating anyway because an answer didn't come that very instant. Today, perseverance has a different meaning. Through working the Twelve Steps and relying on my Higher Power, perseverance now means working through daily struggles with the hope of resolution and a brighter tomorrow, trusting my Higher Power to remove my impatience and replace it with the willingness I need to see that working through struggles is a part of recovery, and in his time, the answers will come. Giving in to daily struggles means I could miss my miracle that could be just five minutes away.

JANUARY 18

"At this point, we learned we could 'act as if.' This didn't mean we were to be dishonestly pious or pretend we believed in God when we didn't. It meant we were free to set aside theological arguments and examine the idea of spiritual power in light of our own desperate need for help with our lives."

—The Twelve Steps and Twelve Traditions of Overeaters Anonymous, 2nd ed., p. 13

I came to OA through AA, where I had been struggling, miserable, and unable to work the program; I simply didn't believe anything could restore me to sanity from my eating and self-harming behavior. Once I had admitted that I was powerless over food, the above quote helped me to take Step Two and move on. Yes, I was absolutely desperate. I could stop being logical, forget my prejudices about the word "God," and "act as if" a power greater than myself was working in my life. "Acting as if" enabled me to start trusting that I would be okay, that I could get through the days without eating compulsively or hurting myself. I don't know what I trust in precisely, but it doesn't matter; I have faith that it works.

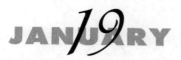

JANUARY 19

"I Put My Hand in Yours ... and together ..."
—*Beyond Our Wildest Dreams*, p. 207

I was alone, and I knew it. I was and am an odd duck—intelligent, yet lacking common sense and tact. I was angry at God. I felt cursed. I ate and ate and ate.

Then came the miracle of program. There my weaknesses were assets. They made me a member. Amazing! I felt understood for the first time. That was the beginning. With fellow compulsive eaters, I daily put down the food and walked the walk of recovery. I reached out my hand, knowing that together we could do what we could never do alone.

In the rooms of OA, I learned the lesson of the AA pioneers: There is a God, and I am not God. In those rooms, I gradually experienced all the promises the Big Book describes. In those rooms, I am home. Today and every day, I am grateful to the God of my understanding that I was desperate enough to reach out and blessed enough to find the hand of OA reaching back.

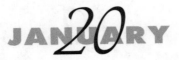

"'Tain't worthwhile to wear a day all out before it comes."

—Sarah Orne Jewett as quoted in *For Today*, p. 182

This quote speaks to me from *For Today* every June 30th. I always have to stop, chuckle to myself, and thank my Higher Power for the reminder (whether I like it or not). It reminds me to take one day at a time, to have a plan, then to turn the day over to my Higher Power's care and trust him for the outcome. This way of living never lets me down! I can get so wrapped up in how I think a day should turn out that by the time it is over, I've missed it! That's why OA tells us to stay in the moment. Yesterday is the past, tomorrow our future, today our present—a present from my Higher Power to be enjoyed one minute at a time. I am learning to stop and smell the roses, take notice of my surroundings, and have gratitude. I have so much living to do today, now that I'm not just surviving in a food fog. OA is teaching me to slow down, breathe deeply, pray like crazy, and trust. I can trust my Higher Power, the Principles of OA, and myself because I am becoming trustworthy. Keep coming back!

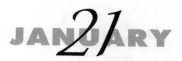

JANUARY 21

*"There is no one right way to do Step Eleven. 'Keep it simple'
is a good slogan to apply here. Remembering that our goal is to
develop a closer conscious contact with God, prayer is simply
what we do when we talk with our Higher Power."*

—The Twelve Steps and Twelve Traditions of Overeaters
Anonymous, 2nd ed., p. 77

When I first got abstinent, my sponsor shared with me that
she writes out her problems and concerns at the end of the
day and puts them in her God box so that she can get a good
night's sleep. The idea, she said, is to let God do the worrying.

I made a big God box and started putting my Tenth Step
in it at bedtime. Then I found myself writing "God notes"
throughout the day and shoving them in my pocket until I
got home to put them in the box. These notes often take the
form of appreciation; gratitude; desires to improve myself; and
requests for a different view when worry, anger, resentment,
confusion, or disappointment take over my thinking. My
prayers bring me closer to God, and my trust in him grows.
God continues to transform my life and my relationships as I
continue, one day at a time, to stuff little pieces of paper into
my oatmeal carton.

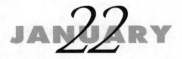

JANUARY 22

"By trying to control others through manipulation and direct force, we had hurt our loved ones. When we tried to control ourselves, we wound up demoralized. Even when we succeeded, it wasn't enough to make us happy."

—*The Twelve Steps and Twelve Traditions of Overeaters Anonymous*, 2nd ed., p. 6

When eating compulsively, I focused on other people's problems. It took the focus off me and created a false sense of power. People couldn't manage their lives without me. "Fixing" other people gave me a false sense of security, much as the huge amount of food seemed to blur all my fears. I believed that this power made people admire, respect, and appreciate me. However, I did not admire, respect, or appreciate myself.

The insanity was in trying to play God for everyone else, then bowing to the god of compulsive overeating when I was alone.

Today, neither food nor control keeps the fears away.

For today, I choose not to do for others what they can do for themselves. I seek God's will, make sure my affairs are in order, and turn the outcome of my life and others' lives over to my Higher Power.

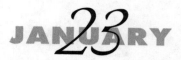

JANUARY 23

"We became willing to start fresh with our Higher Power ... asking ourselves what, exactly, we needed and wanted God to be to us and to do for us."

—*The Twelve Steps and Twelve Traditions of Overeaters Anonymous*, 2nd ed., p. 14

What do I need from my Higher Power? First, I need his protection from the food. I have no other defense against it. Second, I ask for specific, daily direction in my life. I may have to wait an hour, a day, maybe even a week, but I get the direction I seek if I stand still and listen. If I receive no direction, I discover later that my Higher Power needed me to stand still either to protect me from going in the wrong direction or to keep me out of the way so things could unfold according to his greater plans.

I feel comforted to know that he will protect me, even from myself, and that he protects us all and wants what is best for us. My Higher Power knows what is best for me, and turning the direction of my life over to him gives me the freedom and the serenity that are the cornerstones of my program.

Thank you, God, for taking away my obsessions and fears and for directing my life in alignment with your greater plan.

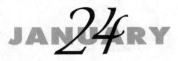

*"Once we took the action and saw it work, we began to believe.
Then we tried other suggestions, and our lives began to be
transformed."*

—The Twelve Steps and Twelve Traditions of Overeaters
Anonymous, 2nd ed., p. 15

My cultural heritage is one of religious, hardworking, and
determined individuals. I learned that if you pray intently,
work diligently, and wait long enough, you can accomplish
anything. However, in the war with food I was a casualty.
The same ten pounds that used to be a battle every six to
nine months was now every two weeks … ten days of starving
followed by four days to regain.

I am a do-it-yourself-er. A pattern, recipe, or creative idea
sets my mind, fingers, and feet in motion. Why wait until
tomorrow when I can start today? (Actually, yesterday is
better.) Here were the Twelve Steps and the Tools. "Just do
it," I was told. I had two textbooks, a phone list, and a sponsor.
My stronghold had a new shipment of arms and reinforcement
of troops. My battleground was the kitchen. The answers to
life are not in the refrigerator or pantry. That was the problem.
Today I live in the answer—the Steps and the Tools. I changed
residence, and the problem went away.

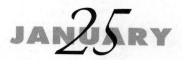

JANUARY 25

"Before we joined the OA Fellowship, our prayers for help might have gone unanswered simply because we were never meant to face this disease in isolation."

—*The Twelve Steps and Twelve Traditions of Overeaters Anonymous,* 2nd ed., p. 14

I was one of those people who prayed regularly for God to remove the fat and allow me to continue overeating. I prayed for the day to be different, not understanding the concept that taking the first bite triggered the disease. I also ate secretly, making sure everyone was out of the house so that I could eat. Today OA offers me the opportunity to be with fellow sufferers who know the pain that excess food has caused. OA offers me recovery from compulsive overeating. I do not need to live in isolation any longer because there are people who understand my disease. What a miracle! I no longer need to isolate myself, as I have come to believe in a Power greater than myself, and I share the camaraderie of fellow compulsive overeaters.

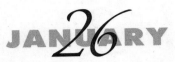

"... praying only for knowledge of His will for us ..."
—Step Eleven

"I don't need much, God. If I could just get to my perfect weight, my life would be perfect." Such was my belief when I arrived at OA. I didn't know this belief would leave my mind battling daily with the food and losing, that my relationships would still be a mess while thoughts of food engulfed my mind, or that my life would still be unmanageable.

Too often, even after years of recovery, I forget that God does not need instructions from me on how to run my life. God knows all my problems, pains, fears, and the inane solutions I often plot in my mind. I need only recall that many years of my best thinking brought me to OA.

No, God does not need a task list from me.

For today I will remember to let an infinite Higher Power enrich my life and broaden my horizons with his will, rather than shortchanging myself with the finite limits of my own human vision.

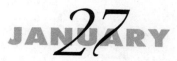
"Abstinence is the most important thing in my life without exception."

—*Lifeline Sampler*, p. 3

I became abstinent when working the Steps and using the Tools. I found physical recovery and a life filled with emotion. During that time, OA members were debating whether abstinence or God was the most important thing in recovery.

I decided to accept the gift of abstinence and maintain it. If abstinence is a gift, then who is the giver? Obviously, it is my loving Higher Power. If I refuse to do the footwork to accept and maintain the gift, then I negate the love my Higher Power has for me. In refusing the gift and denying the love, I cannot say that my relationship with my Higher Power is the most important thing in my life. In fact, the opposite would be true.

I now have no problem believing that abstinence is the most important thing in my life without exception. For me, it can work no other way because this belief expresses the physical and emotional foundation of OA, and it embodies the spiritual essence of it.

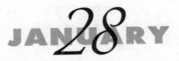
*"I keep an open mind to having an open mind; the possibilities
are endless."*

—*For Today*, p. 237

When I came into these rooms, I was absolutely closed-minded regarding religious matters. But I soon realized two things: religious matters were not the same as a spiritual experience; and a spiritual experience was absolutely necessary if I were to survive this disease of compulsive overeating. Once I did the footwork and became willing to open myself to a spiritual experience, it happened. I didn't make it happen, but I did allow it to happen by setting up inviting conditions: quiet time for meditation, writing, and prayer.

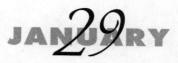
"You are kidding yourself if you think 'just one bite' will 'bring back the good old days' or make some bad situation better or easier to live with."

—*A Lifetime of Abstinence: One Day at a Time*, p. 5

Even after more than five years in this program, food thoughts still pop into my mind when I feel stressed, frustrated, or depressed. Although I would love to have complete freedom from such thoughts, I'm learning to accept that I have the mind of a compulsive overeater, a mind that automatically associates feelings of discomfort with the siren song of food. The quote above reminds me that no matter how strong my desire to eat may be, it's never the food that I really want; therefore, eating won't make me feel better. If I am upset and craving food, I really need to connect with my Higher Power, to spend some quiet time by myself, or to talk to a caring friend. Thus, recovery has taught me that even though I may think like a compulsive overeater, I don't have to act like one.

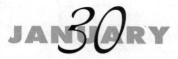

"Our true insanity could be seen in the fact that we kept right on trying to find comfort in excess food, long after it began to cause us misery."

—*The Twelve Steps and Twelve Traditions of Overeaters Anonymous*, 2nd ed., p. 11

I can remember when a little food gave me comfort or relief. That was many years ago. The quest to relive that feeling resulted in bigger and more frequent binges. Eventually, I began to see that this may not be normal—but insane? I wasn't convinced.

Was it insane to eat to a point of such fullness that exploding might have been a relief? To purge myself with laxatives so the binge wouldn't have time to cause a weight gain? To eat so fast and furiously as to cause cuts on my lips and inside my mouth, and still to keep eating until the bag was empty? To try starving myself for a few days after a binge, almost as a punishment for what I had done? To eat the substances that caused me migraine headaches and rage outbursts? Was it insane to stop living in return for nonstop eating?

I must answer yes to all of the above. I am convinced.

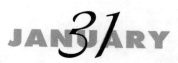

"Just for today."

—program slogan

"Just for today" is one of the program slogans that works for me. It is even better than "one day at a time" because that suggests another day coming. Sometimes, today is as much as I can handle. As *Just for Today* says, "I can do something for one day that would appall me if I felt that I had to keep it up for a lifetime." At times, I have had to say to myself, "Only four, three, two more hours until I go to bed, close my eyes, don't have to talk to one more person or do one more thing." It is a sublimely peaceful feeling to reach the end of that one day, to be finished.

"Just for today" also helps me avoid the notion that I have some space from my disease if I have a few days, weeks, or months of abstinence in a row. When the days run together and I get farther from my last compulsive bite, I can begin to think that I have somehow "made it" or that I've reached a safe distance from my disease. Nothing could be further from the truth. I am as close to taking that first compulsive bite today as I was on the day I came into program if I am not living in the present and aware that I am a compulsive overeater. "Just for today" reminds me that today is all I have.

FEBRUARY 1

"Came to believe that a Power greater than ourselves could restore us to sanity."
—Step Two

After twenty-one years in OA, I'm beginning to understand Step Two as a "process." When I began OA, God was in my life, but I didn't understand God's part in restoring me to sanity. I struggled for years trying to do it myself: making and breaking diets, planning rewards and punishments, setting goals and never reaching them—always failing.

Not until I began to let go of my old beliefs and open my mind to new ways of thinking did I begin to understand what "came to believe that a Power greater than ourselves" meant. It meant that God is greater than me, that he loves me enough to restore me to sanity if I ask each day, and that I can trust him to do it. My work is to give my eating to him each day. His work is to restore me to sane living and eating. The results are his, not mine. Now I'm making a shift from a me-centered life to a God-centered one.

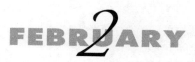

FEBRUARY 2

"For an honest, balanced view of myself, I take a few moments in which I free my mind of everything except God's love for me."

—*For Today*, p. 153

One of the hardest things for me when meditating was emptying my mind of the "mind chatter" that crowded out contemplative thoughts. That changed when I read this quotation. I love to meditate to this quotation. I visualize God's love enveloping me like a warm glow. Sometimes I visualize a white light surrounding me. I can then empty my mind of everything except God's love for me, leaving me with a sense of well-being for myself and the world. Problems and difficulties melt away. I feel intensely grateful for being alive and for all the good things in my life. It's not that I don't have problems anymore; it's just that I realize that having problems and overcoming them is what life is about. Why else are we here?

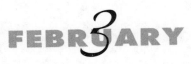

FEBRUARY 3

"Coming to believe was something that happened as we began taking actions that others told us had worked for them. Whether we believed these actions would work for us didn't seem to matter. Once we took the action and saw it work, we began to believe."

— *The Twelve Steps and Twelve Traditions of Overeaters Anonymous*, 2nd ed., p. 15

This is one of the secrets of the OA program: "We cannot think ourselves into good action, but we can act ourselves into good thinking." Willingness to follow the suggestions of the program leads us to healing the wreckage of our lives and the ravages of this disease.

I experienced the miracle of abstinence because I asked someone to sponsor me; I designed a practical, nourishing food plan; and I committed daily to following my plan and calling my sponsor.

I experienced the healing bonds of fellowship because I attended meetings regularly and became involved in service.

I experienced a spiritual awakening because I put all my doubts and fears aside and placed my reliance on a Higher Power of my own understanding instead of on my distorted self-will.

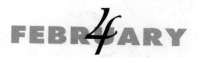

FEBRUARY 4

"And if it can happen for me, it can happen for you."
—*Lifeline Sampler*, p. 317

"Are you willing to go to any lengths?" asked my sponsor.

"I am," I answered. "I ring you every day, I pray, I go to meetings, I write, I'm doing everything you say, so why can't I just get abstinent?" My sponsor replied that not only did I have to do all these things, I also had to put down the food. I had to stop eating compulsively. She promised that if I put down the food and picked up the Steps, eventually the desire to eat compulsively would leave me. And it has. One day at a time, for more than nine years, I've been almost totally free of the desire to eat compulsively.

It seems that the less I overeat, the less I feel like overeating. In the early days I felt like overeating all the time. My sponsor said, "Don't eat, no matter what"—and I didn't. These days I rarely feel like overeating. Through "putting down the food and picking up the Steps," the desire to overeat compulsively has been lifted.

Thank you, God. Thank you, OA. If it can happen for me and for countless others, it can happen for you too.

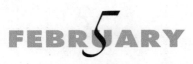

FEBRUARY 5

"Clearly, if we were to be restored to sanity, we had to find a Power greater than ourselves."

—*The Twelve Steps and Twelve Traditions of Overeaters Anonymous*, 2nd ed., p. 12

For someone as impulsive and driven to find relief as I was, sanity took many forms: waiting instead of acting, looking for the positive in a situation, feelings of satisfaction when the action fell short of the intention, and learning to be aware of my compulsion and think it through.

When I relied on my wits alone, I used all my energy to make things happen. Too often I met with frustration, disappointment, and feelings of failure or self-pity, which led me back to the food.

The Higher Power I found in Overeaters Anonymous revealed a more peaceful approach to living. He enabled me to begin asking for help, contemplate my options, and anticipate the effect of my actions on others.

I began to trust in this Higher Power, trust my instincts, and, ultimately, trust other people. Now my faith in that Power reveals itself in the smallest decisions during my day.

I feel a calmness and a confidence that produce realistic expectations under adversity. Now that's sanity.

FEBR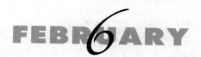ARY

"Avoid dwelling on pleasant memories associated with certain foods or thoughts about how good a particular food might taste."
—*A Lifetime of Abstinence: One Day at a Time,* p. 5

I enlarged this pamphlet and cut it into squares. Each piece of paper had one suggestion on it. I put them up, one at a time, in a corner of my bathroom mirror and read them over and over until they became recorded in my mind.

After eleven years of contented abstinence, I'm still using those suggestions, especially the one about not allowing myself to think about how a certain food might taste. It still works to keep food thoughts from getting into my mind and developing into obsessions.

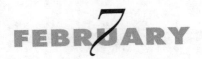

FEBRUARY 7

*"Sought through prayer and meditation to improve our
conscious contact with God ..."*

—Step Eleven

Unconscious eating is one of the ways I express my lack
of conscious contact with God. Eating is a habit and a
compulsion.

When frightened or angry, I often find myself in the kitchen
without being completely conscious of what I'm doing. While
preparing meals, I often find myself starting to put something
in my mouth without thinking. I hardly know I'm doing it.

That is why I must stay in the present, aware of my actions
and emotions, particularly around food. Meditation at some
time during the day gives me practice in concentrated thought:
the experience of being completely present.

Before I approach food or food preparation, it helps me to
remember the first three Steps and to say the Serenity Prayer.

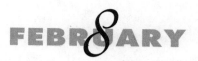

FEBRUARY 8

"We, as individuals, are fully self-supporting only when we do what we can, when we can, giving back some of the help we have been given in OA."

—*The Twelve Steps and Twelve Traditions of Overeaters Anonymous*, 2nd ed., p. 135

This is a beautiful paradox for living, for happiness, for control over my eating addiction. I had wanted to be self-supporting and self-reliant by using the shrewd methods of financial planning. I had wanted to keep my few resources, so I would have plenty to provide for my needs. But the "wise and experienced" ones in OA tell me I can do so only when I get into the heart of the program, which is to do and to give. I don't have to do this to extremes, only "what and when I can." My eating habits and character changed when I adopted this philosophy.

Would any amount of money or service repay this loving Fellowship that has saved my life? I think not. Before I recognized the importance of this program, I resented being asked for monetary contributions. It was when I saw that this Fellowship is not "me" and "them," but "us," that I found I could do more in both service and money than I had pretended I could.

Any amount of "giving back some of the help I have received" gives me unmeasured serenity and energy. It gives me the creativeness to do "what I can, when I can" in a true spirit of gratitude.

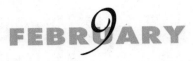

FEBRUARY 9

"*No matter how long we abstain from eating compulsively and no matter how adept we become at facing life, we will always have these abnormal tendencies.*"

—*The Twelve Steps and Twelve Traditions of Overeaters Anonymous*, 2nd ed., p. 4

While I am in recovery, abstaining and working the Steps, my disease is with me, waiting for an opportunity to tempt me back into self-destruction. Long-term abstinence and recovery give me good habits to fall back on in times of pain and exhaustion, but they are not enough.

I have seen too many people with years of abstinence in OA leave this program and fall into serious relapse and weight gain. These were compulsive overeaters who worked serious programs and who had experienced fully the freedom, joy, and serenity of recovery.

Why did they fall from grace? Because they have a chronic, incurable disease that requires daily application of this program and conscious surrender to God. Circumstances in their lives distracted them from the knowledge that abstinence was their most pressing concern.

Self-will, ego, and denial will always lead me back into self-destruction with food.

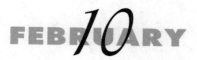

FEBRUARY 10

"Entrust yourself and your abstinence to a Power greater than yourself."

—*A Lifetime of Abstinence: One Day at a Time*, p. 4

The stress of attempting to trust myself when my disease was rampant was like trying to push a rope up a tree—impossible. I'm grateful that today I have a Higher Power I can trust to guide me in honesty and truth.

I no longer have to depend on my own unsteady willpower. I now live in God's will, which I receive through the Step Eleven prayer, and I can rest in God's love through my fellow recovering OA members.

When fear strikes my heart, I remember that fear and faith cannot dwell in the same place at the same time. When I fear myself or other people, places, or things, it reminds me to concentrate on faith. For me, that means more surrender, more prayer, and more meditation. I consciously and gratefully receive more of God's love through family, friends, and the Fellowship.

I still make mistakes, but I no longer fear my thoughts, my actions, or my disease because I trust my Higher Power.

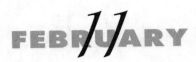

FEBRUARY 11

"Those who cannot remember the past are condemned to repeat it."
—George Santayana as quoted in *For Today*, p. 331

I was an unhappy compulsive overeater my entire life, always going on diets and then getting heavier afterwards. "Tomorrow," I would say, "I will lose weight," but tomorrow I forgot yesterday's misery. My father and brother both died at age fifty-seven of heart attacks, and I was convinced I would die at the age of fifty-seven also. At age forty-eight, I had a heart attack and bypass surgery to move blood past the arteries that my compulsive eating had blocked. I lost weight but soon forgot the pain; I gained even more weight a year after the surgery. I thought my life was hopeless.

A friend dragged me to an OA meeting, and I started on a path that changed my life. OA taught me how to change "tomorrow" one day at a time, to change my old habits, to remember the past. I gave up over ninety pounds, and the miracle is that I have kept them off for over two years. I just celebrated my fifty-eighth birthday. Today I don't forget the past. I now focus on being abstinent and alive.

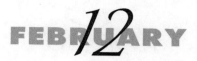

"Recovery began for most of us when we got out of isolation and into an OA group. Here we discovered we were not alone."

—*The Twelve Steps and Twelve Traditions of Overeaters Anonymous*, 2nd ed., p. 91

There's something about this Fellowship of individuals that has completely changed my life.

I think the spirituality of OA comes from the comforting word "we." I'm not alone. I used to find my comfort in food, but it was a lonely, sad kind of comfort. Now my comfort is in this Fellowship.

There's much love in this program. Even if I feel tired and cranky when I walk into a meeting, smiles and hugs greet me. The honest sharing, holding of hands, and praying transform and energize me.

When I can't make a meeting, I can make a phone call. When I can't make a phone call, I can send an email or write a letter to another OA member.

I'm part of a "we." In this wonderful program I've found love and understanding beyond my wildest dreams. Thank God for OA.

"Those who are prone to stuff themselves with food that makes their bodies unsightly are refusing the food that satisfies and soothes the unhappy soul within."

—*Overeaters Anonymous*, 3rd ed., p. 205

It took a couple of shocks to get me to accept the idea that spiritual weakness was part of my disease. After all, I had always believed in a Higher Power I called God and had attended church almost every Sunday of my life. So I took a bit of offense to this quotation and, even more so, to my first sponsor's statement that it was obvious that food was my god.

However, when I faced the many ways I had given food power over my life, I started to pray for forgiveness. I had not only used food to comfort, console, or reward me, but to give me energy and to help me sleep. As a result of my eleven-year journey in OA, I now see my Higher Power as a very personal and loving God, there to guide and direct me if I just open myself to him and listen. He has done so much more for me than food could ever do. Indeed, this spiritual link is essential to my day-by-day abstinence from compulsive overeating.

"The Twelfth Step invites us to continue the journey one day at a time for the rest of our lives. We need to keep moving forward in recovery, keep developing our spiritual consciousness, if we are to remain spiritually awake and fully alive."

—*The Twelve Steps and Twelve Traditions of Overeaters Anonymous*, 2nd ed., p. 82

Through the practice of the Twelve Steps I have been awakened spiritually. And by continuing to practice these Principles throughout my day, I may remain free of the bondage to food. As it says in the Big Book of Alcoholics Anonymous, I believe I have a daily reprieve contingent upon the maintenance of my spiritual condition.

I am truly grateful that a Higher Power has removed from me the obsession to eat and replaced it with the willingness to use the Tools of this program, which enable me to live life on life's terms. I trust that no matter what happens in my life today, picking up the food will not take away the pain or make me "feel better." I have come to realize that nothing happens in God's world by mistake. The best thing I can do today is get on with the next thing that's in front of me, and all things will pass.

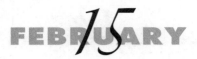

FEBRUARY 15

"Surrender, then, is an unconscious event. It is not willed by the individual. It can occur only when one becomes involved with one's unconscious mind in a set of circumstances that signal the undeniable need for an external greater power. The definition of surrender can be understood only when all its unconscious ramifications and true inner meaning are glimpsed. Observed by others, such an individual manifests an inner calm and a 'live and let live' attitude."

—*Overeaters Anonymous*, 3rd ed., p. 202

I felt relieved when I read this passage. It meant I could not control my surrender process. I could only be willing and do the footwork. By attending OA meetings, calling other OA members, reading, writing, and working the Steps, I became teachable and put myself in a set of circumstances that signaled the undeniable need for an external greater power. I began to see that my going on a diet every Monday, New Year's Day, and birthday didn't work and never would—but OA might. For OA to work, I had to be willing to let go, or surrender, and take the first three Steps.

About thirteen months after my first meeting, surrender happened one July morning. I just quit. I got sick and tired of being sick and tired. I called an abstinent program friend, asked her what she did, and adopted a plan of eating. I've been imperfectly abstinent ever since.

I made that phone call more than twenty years ago, and what worked then still works today. I'm grateful to OA and pray for continued surrender, abstinence, and a wonderful life, one day at a time.

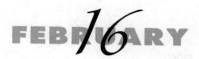

> *"That these didn't make us happy was surely due to the fact*
> *that we were fat (or felt we were). If we could just get to the*
> *perfect weight, life would be wonderful."*
>
> —*The Twelve Steps and Twelve Traditions of Overeaters*
> *Anonymous,* 2nd ed., p. 5

I became abstinent after my first meeting and was a normal weight after six months. I ignored the emotional and spiritual parts of the program, thinking I might get to them eventually. I lost my abstinence, but started abstaining again and knew that recovery had to be more than a diet or a "normal" weight. None of my problems went away when I was a normal weight. I thought normal-weight people had no problems, and I envied them. Now I realize that "normal" people deal with difficulties rather than pushing them down with food. With my Higher Power's help, I too can recover.

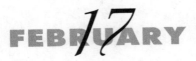

FEBRUARY 17

*"For our group purpose there is but one ultimate authority—
a loving God as He may express Himself in our group
conscience...."*

—Tradition Two

I had a small amount of religious training when I was young, and I thought I knew what I needed to know about God and prayer. My biggest stumbling blocks in program were that my concept of God didn't apply when it came to compulsive overeating, and my concept of prayer didn't include anything personal. Suddenly the Steps were asking me to turn my will and my life over to something greater than myself, but nothing in my religious or intellectual thought fit. The idea of making this Power a book or a tree or my sponsor didn't seem reasonable. Then I heard someone refer to "a loving God as expressed in the Second Tradition." I realized that whatever I wanted my God to be was all right, as long as that Power was loving. Nothing else mattered. I imagined a benevolent friend, and my intellectual and religious arguments disappeared.

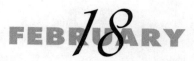

FEBRUARY 18

> *"Real humility about our character defects carries with it acceptance."*
>
> —*The Twelve Steps and Twelve Traditions of Overeaters Anonymous*, 2nd ed., p. 53

I think of my personality characteristics as being something similar to a sound system. When the characteristics are moderate, the volume control is in the center. When the characteristics are way out of proportion, they become character defects. Take self-esteem, for example. If the volume is too high, I am practicing false pride. If the volume is too low, I am suffering from self-esteem problems.

I have to acknowledge, if I am humble, that my character defects may never be removed, but they can be tempered. They can be moderated by my Higher Power as long as I take my hands off the volume control. Humility means I know these things are going to keep showing up, and I get to keep asking God to put me back in balance.

> *"Those of us who live this program don't simply carry the message; we are the message. Each day that we live well, we are well, and we embody the joy of recovery, which attracts others who want what we've found in OA."*
>
> —The Twelve Steps and Twelve Traditions of Overeaters Anonymous, 2nd ed., pp. 86–87

When I am in recovery, I am better able to share the OA message with the world. My thoughts are clearer to me, and I can live my life according to the Steps and Traditions. I listen carefully to the messages of others and tell my fellow OA members what I was like and what I have done to save my life.

Staying abstinent and working the spiritual and emotional parts of this program are the only ways I can survive this deadly disease. When I depend on my Higher Power, my sponsor's wisdom, and the meetings I attend, my recovery grows daily. Using the Tools keeps me focused on living to the best of my ability.

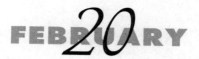
"What we do have to offer is … a Fellowship in which we find and share the healing power of love."

> —*The Twelve Steps and Twelve Traditions of Overeaters Anonymous*, 2nd ed., p. 1

When I entered the Twelve Step program, I was broken, bleeding, discouraged, debauched, bloated, and hating myself. Then came my first ray of hope: "We will love you until you can love yourself!" Yes (praise God), this miracle has come true. I love and respect myself today. I had been badly buffeted by life, including other compulsions and major illnesses. However, my health as a total person is much improved. Love from others in OA and from my Higher Power has healed me. I have learned to accept myself without judgment, as other OA members accept and love me. I, too, can now reach out in Overeaters Anonymous and let love pass through me to heal others. To every newcomer I say, "We will love you until you can love yourself."

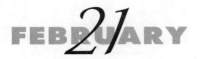

FEBRUARY 21

"In OA, we learn that our recovery comes to us through the Principles of the program, not through personalities."

—*The Twelve Steps and Twelve Traditions of Overeaters Anonymous*, 2nd ed., p. 166

We are taught, through loving acts of tact and kindness under difficult circumstances, that we are given far more than a normal body size as a result of taking OA's Twelve Steps and remaining abstinent.

Since recovery in OA is a transformational journey, conflict with others is inevitable, and often unavoidable. The shame and low self-esteem that prey on us afterwards are the voice of our disease, calling us back.

Today, I can view my differences with others, both personal and philosophical, as opportunities to identify and overcome my knee-jerk reactions to the world in which I live. I can tolerate the feelings and sidestep the temptation to abbreviate my discomfort by speaking or acting inappropriately, knowing that a short-term "fix" won't work for someone like me.

I pray that I may always seek God's help to move towards the most harmonious relations with others, knowing that my abstinence may hinge on my reaction to life in this moment. The OA Principles will always lead me in that direction.

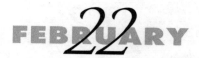

FEBRUARY 22

"OA doesn't tell us we have to believe in God—only that 'a Power greater than ourselves could restore us to sanity.'"

—*The Twelve Steps and Twelve Traditions of Overeaters Anonymous*, 2nd ed., p. 12

My concept of a Higher Power has changed, just as I have changed. I am not the same person I once was. I had worshipped God in church, so it was easy to return to that setting. However, after a few years, I realized that I no longer believed God was big enough to restore me to sanity. He worked in the lives of everyone else, but not in mine.

My sponsor said I was suffering from "tiny God syndrome." She suggested that I borrow her Higher Power while I was trying to define my own. If that was not big enough, I could take all the Higher Powers from everyone at our big meeting. It reminded me of taking little pieces of clay from here and there until I had a big pile.

Every time I thought of something big, I came up with something bigger. Finally, I realized that when the sun shines, it doesn't shine in just one spot, and that maybe God's love could be that big.

"Just for today I will have a quiet half hour all by myself and relax. During this half hour, sometime, I will try to get a better perspective on my life."

—Just For Today

When I was new in OA, my sponsor suggested that, at a minimum, I give God the first fifteen minutes of each morning as my Step Eleven. She said that if I did, God would take care of the rest of the day, including my abstinence. I did that minimum, and my life improved. Soon it became obvious that I needed the willingness to do more than the minimum—in every aspect of my recovery. As a result, I learned to carry Step Eleven from the sacred space of my morning into every aspect of my day: shopping, working, cooking, eating, and even standing in line at the post office.

The more we do, the more we get back. As I began, to the very best of my ability, to practice spiritual Principles in all my affairs, miracles of healing began to happen. I became eager to try everything my sponsor and the Big Book suggested. Abstinence became easy, and I became hungry for a Principle-based life. The miracles kept happening and have never stopped. It really does work when we work it!

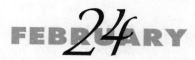

"The illusions I had as a compulsive overeater were at the root of my illness....

When exposed to the bright light of reality these ideas—my old illusions—crumble into dust and blow away."

—For Today, p. 134

I carried the illusions I brought with me to this program for many years. For example, if I were a "good girl," life would bring me no pain; when I married, I would be taken care of; I could control people, places, and things; being thin would solve all my problems; if I had enough willpower, I could stop eating.

When I came into Overeaters Anonymous, these illusions were exposed to the bright light of the Twelve Steps, and gradually they lost their hold over me. OA gave me the courage, hope, and clarity to face my life, one day at a time, without eating compulsively. Today I believe that living in reality carries with it the widest spectrum of feelings and challenges. When I keep the Twelve Steps close at hand, I have a chance to experience the promises and gifts of this program.

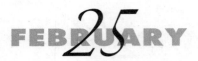

FEBRUARY 25

"We ... realize the futility of continuing to blame others for our eating behaviors and unmanageable lives."

—*The Twelve Steps and Twelve Traditions of Overeaters Anonymous,* 2nd ed., p. 40

Ouch! This idea hits hard. For many years, I transferred blame for my uncontrolled eating and unmanageable life to the villain of the day. Depending on the situation that resulted in my overeating, the villain could be my parents, sister, husband, children, employer, coworkers, friends, enemies. In other words, anyone or anything that stood between me and my desires could cause me to eat. Today, I acknowledge that eating compulsively is my choice, not an outcome imposed on me by some external force.

I know today that my Higher Power will help me make reasonable choices about all aspects of my life if I only ask. Thanks to the presence of a Higher Power in my life, I am no longer at the mercy of multiple dictators.

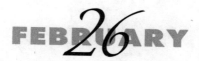

"Ours is a spiritual program, not a religious one. We have no creeds or doctrines, only our own experiences of recovery."

—*The Twelve Steps and Twelve Traditions of Overeaters Anonymous, 2nd ed., p. 12*

I was never a religious person, or even a spiritual one for that matter. When I first came to OA, I had difficulty with the idea of a Higher Power. Honestly, it scared me. I wanted to believe, but I just didn't know how. It was only by talking with several members who openly shared their ideas of a Higher Power that I was able to open my own mind. I did something I couldn't do for thirty years: I came to believe in a Power greater than myself. The fact that OA is a spiritual program, and not a religious one, is why I am still here. Today I believe in a Power greater than myself, a loving, caring Higher Power that I define in my own words.

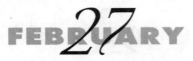
"Unity does not mean uniformity. In OA, we learn we can disagree with other people on important issues and still be supportive friends."

—*The Twelve Steps and Twelve Traditions of Overeaters Anonymous*, 2nd ed., p. 95

Service in Overeaters Anonymous has taught me many things. Perhaps the most important is that I can love and respect someone with a different point of view. We are members of the same Fellowship; we share the same compulsion. We are both trying to do what is best for OA, and we can "agree to disagree." Through OA I've learned that we can have different viewpoints on an issue without jeopardizing our friendship. Just because someone disagrees with me doesn't mean that person doesn't love me or want my friendship. I don't have to take it personally. Our group conscience decides an issue. If I don't agree with the decision by group conscience, I can nevertheless learn to live with it. I trust that others also have the good of OA as a whole in mind, and I can learn something. I can learn that not only are there other views than mine, but that they may be right.

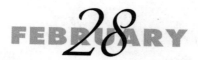
"Real humility about our character defects carries with it acceptance."

—*The Twelve Steps and Twelve Traditions of Overeaters Anonymous*, 2nd ed., p. 53

One of the most wonderful gifts I have received in this program is accepting and even loving myself. This new attitude has made it possible for me to take an honest look at the makeup of my character.

In Steps Six and Seven I have learned to deal with my character defects. I know now that I don't have to identify myself with my faults; I can make a mistake but that doesn't mean that I am a mistake.

I can take responsibility for mistakes and character defects by being honest (and not judgmental) with myself and by asking my Higher Power for love and guidance and to help me surrender them to him/her. The change in me, which indeed does occur, has shown me once again that the secret of success lies in surrender.

For today I can ask my Higher Power for awareness of myself, along with the willingness to surrender and to let me be as I am supposed to be.

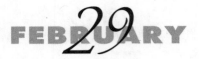

FEBRUARY 29

"The only gift is a portion of thyself."

—Ralph Waldo Emerson as quoted in *For Today*, p. 360

At a recent conference, I saw Step Twelve acted out in all of its glory. My three sponsors, all of whom have years of back-to-back abstinence, were there encouraging, telling others how to do it. They knew that they would probably not hear anything new for themselves. They went only to bring the message of healing to someone who was still suffering.

They are living proof of good health, energy, and normal weight. They are the promises exemplified. Their faces shone with abstinence and the joy of themselves.

As if that were not enough, when we got home, we all attended our regular meeting. The leader of the evening had us share what we had experienced at the conference. That way, everyone got to go.

As we hugged each other goodbye, one of my sponsors was chuckling to herself, "I have to hurry home in case my new sponsee from the conference calls." She just keeps on giving and giving and giving.

I follow my sponsor's example. I am abstinent, healthy, and enjoy my life and everyone in it. I am ready to sponsor. I finally have something to give.

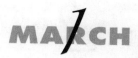

MARCH 1

"Made a decision to turn our will and our lives over to the care of God as we understood Him."
—Step Three

What freedom I've found in knowing that when I work Step Three and turn my will and my life and my food over to my Higher Power, I am no longer powerless. The Big Book tells me that a new power flows in. I am then empowered to make healthy choices. Abstinence is no longer the struggle it was when I was trying to abstain by willpower alone.

Allowing this new power to flow in constantly and consistently throughout this day, I see that cravings are not commands, and relapse is never inevitable. I can do this. I can move through this day abstinent and free. I now affirm, "Abstinence is the easiest thing I have ever done."

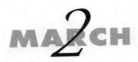

MARCH 2

*"Once we compulsive eaters truly take the Third Step,
we cannot fail to recover."*

> —*The Twelve Steps and Twelve Traditions of Overeaters
> Anonymous,* 2nd ed., p. 23

After telling my story at meetings, I get flurries of phone calls from old and new members asking for the "inside scoop" on how I really did it. It's not just the seventy-three pounds I released; people want to know about the serenity, what keeps me centered and calm despite hair-raising personal experiences in my life. What made the program's tenets click now, finally?

Simple: the Third Step corresponds to the Principle of faith. Once we truly make the leap to believe, no matter what, that a Power greater than ourselves will restore us to sanity and will take care of every other issue in our lives as well, we cannot ever fail to recover, and the compulsion to binge disappears. It has to happen! That Power, I now know, has always been there for me, like a bridge waiting to be crossed. It's so simple that most of us believe there must be more to it than that, some other trick or secret.

There are no secrets, no magic. Anyone can have what I have. I've been cornered, trapped. The gate to freedom has closed behind me. I looked inward and there was honesty. I looked outward and there was hope. I looked up and there was faith.

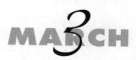

MARCH 3

"I picked up the phone; my life changed and OA's future abruptly took a new direction."

—*Beyond Our Wildest Dreams,* p. 85

What a simple program we have. Just reaching out to each other makes our lives change and affects the future of the meetings. I have had many telephone calls that have been just the "right" message I needed at the time I was most wanting a helping hand. Often I called someone because my desire to overeat was strong, and just the act of dialing the phone changed the emotion from negative to the release of energy that can start meetings, begin new intergroups, and even save lives. I am grateful that the Tools of telephone, anonymity, service, and meetings all work together in recovery.

"Always to extend the hand and heart of OA to all who share my compulsion; for this I am responsible" (OA Responsibility Pledge).

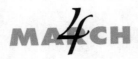

MARCH 4

"... as we understood Him ..."
—Step Eleven

Today I am not burdened by my or anyone else's preconceptions about a Higher Power. By working the Steps, using the slogans, and taking advantage of the Tools, I have met a power greater than myself that works for me. Prayer and meditation are what I need daily to be the complete and abstinent person that I am.

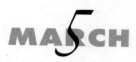

MARCH 5

"A problem is solved and immediately there is hope that an even tougher one will go the same way."

—*For Today*, p. 3

One day as we discussed a difficult relationship problem, my sponsor said, "If you're doing it to please him, you're back in your disease." That statement helped me see that on the emotional side of my recovery, God was rarely my Higher Power. Sometimes my Higher Power was my husband; sometimes it was the immature parts of my personality; sometimes it was people whose acceptance and approval I wanted. These people, including my childish self, had power over me to control my thoughts, feelings, and actions.

I began to see that even though I was physically abstinent, I wasn't emotionally abstinent. I still tried to control things, such as the outcome of events and the behavior and feelings of those around me. Maybe that was why I lacked serenity and my life seemed out of control and overwhelming. I felt discouraged, but the line from *For Today* reassured me, "A problem is solved and immediately there is hope that an even tougher one will go the same way." I began writing my way through the Steps to learn the difference between compulsive emotional behavior and emotional abstinence. Today God helps me to be emotionally abstinent. I do the footwork, and God does for me what I cannot do for myself.

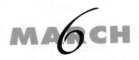

MARCH 6

"*Then I heard about OA on a radio talk show. From that moment on, life has been different.*"

—*Lifeline Sampler*, p. 199

How do I feel reading that? Hearing and responding to that broadcast saved the life of the person who wrote about it. What if there had been no broadcast to hear?

I do not like to think that I have been hiding behind "Do what you can, when you can," but have I been letting myself off too easily from Twelfth Step work?

Could I bring the needs of those who do not know about OA into my prayer and meditation? Should I raise the question of a Twelve Step project at my home group? Is it time to answer telephones?

Getting honest with myself about my eating was the beginning of this great improvement in the quality of my life. What might happen to the quality of my life if I got honest with myself about Step Twelve? What can I do in the next twenty-four hours to reach another sufferer? Making this program better known is partly up to me.

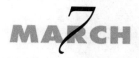

MARCH 7

"Instead of acting on impulse, we pause long enough to learn God's will. Then, instead of resorting to willpower, we relax and reach out to receive help from our Higher Power. All we need to say is 'God, please help me do your will.'"

—The Twelve Steps and Twelve Traditions of Overeaters Anonymous, 2nd ed., p. 23

In my recovery, I am learning to slow down and listen to the voice inside me that is my Higher Power. This presence is always with me, but in the chatter of everyday life and wanting to do things my way, this voice is often drowned out. When I slow down and tune it, I hear it loud and clear. In revisiting the Third Step through these words whenever I need to, I live my recovery. That is a true miracle—to know that through these few words of supplication—let me do your will—I move beyond myself to something greater. It always guides me and is always a gift—because when I ask for willingness to do God's will, I give up control of what I think should happen. I am always surprised.

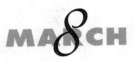

MARCH 8

"We complete our amends for our wrongful actions of the past by changing our actions in the future."

—*The Twelve Steps and Twelve Traditions of Overeaters Anonymous*, 2nd ed., pp. 65–66

Though it can be humbling to apologize for something I've done wrong, it's easy to feel remorse when the pain of a recent mistake is still with me. The test of my commitment to the Ninth Step is if I continue to improve my behavior after the initial feelings of regret have passed.

To amend something means to alter it. To be free of the wreckage of my past, I have to do more than just say I'm sorry when I harm another person. I have to change my behavior. This can be hard and sometimes even disconcerting, particularly when my old behavior patterns and beliefs are stronger than I thought. But continuing to work the Steps moves me through the difficult spots to new experiences of freedom and joy.

The fruits of recovery are great motivators to change, but alongside the hope of a brighter future is the equally powerful consequence of not changing—compulsive eating. If I don't change my thoughts and actions to reduce the harm I do in the future, I will overeat. For me, to overeat is to die.

A life well-lived requires that I continue to change, grow, and clean up the wreckage of my past—and my present. If I do that, my life is better than I could have ever imagined. I thank my Higher Power for OA!

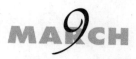

MARCH 9

> *"'Spiritual, emotional, and physical recovery is achieved through living and working the Overeaters Anonymous Twelve Step program.'"*
>
> —*A Lifetime of Abstinence: One Day at a Time,* p. 1

Abstinence, to me, is very simple. It is refraining from compulsive overeating and continuing to work my program. Compulsive overeating is when I wander around my kitchen shoveling food into my mouth unthinkingly. Compulsiveness is when I am not reading, writing, calling, and using the other Tools. Compulsiveness is when I do not use the Steps or talk to my Higher Power.

Abstinence is eating balanced meals, using the OA Tools, practicing the Steps and Traditions, sponsoring, and doing other service. I can binge on veggies, so I do not have a food list that determines my abstinence. Instead, it is an action that undermines my abstinence: eating compulsively—feeding feelings, bingeing, stuffing my face. Recovery is threefold—physical, spiritual, and emotional. If I only count the physical (adhering to a food plan), I miss out on two important parts of recovery.

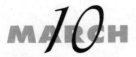

"We find that our Higher Power often leads us through our blunders."

—*The Twelve Steps and Twelve Traditions of Overeaters Anonymous,* 2nd ed., p. 101

If I had my way, I would always walk a straight and smooth path that would lead directly to my goals. My Higher Power seems to have other ideas. Even though the Twelve Step path is well marked, I always seem to wander off on a trail that winds through surprising territory. Turning my will and life over to God as I understand God means I cease demanding perfection of myself, of others, of life. Instead, I relax and enjoy the view on those strange detours in my road. I may feel lost and confused, but God knows the way. Sometimes I try to take shortcuts and wind up hurting myself and others. I make amends and get back on the road. My blunders teach me the pathways that lead to dead ends so I can avoid them in the future. I make many mistakes, but I cannot really lose as long as I keep turning back to the OA Fellowship and the Twelve Steps.

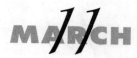

MARCH 11

"Compulsive eating is an illness that cannot be controlled
by willpower. None of us decided to have this disorder."

— *The Twelve Steps and Twelve Traditions of Overeaters
Anonymous*, 2nd ed., p. 4

I find such freedom in this idea. I am not responsible for
having this disease. I don't have to beat myself up for being
a compulsive overeater anymore. I also don't have to waste
time trying to "fix" myself in ways that don't work. Though
sworn by many of my friends to be the answer to their weight
problems, willpower does nothing for my disease. Applying
willpower to this compulsion is like applying an antibiotic to a
viral infection. It will never have any effect.

What does prevail against this disease is working the Steps.
When I really work them, I recover spiritually, emotionally,
and physically. Then I'm able to truly believe what Step One
tells me: I'm not responsible for the disease. I'm not weak
from lack of willpower. I'm strong because I'm fighting it, and
with my Higher Power on my side, there's no way the disease
can win.

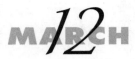

MARCH 12

"*While working toward a healthy body weight, many of us may have been so focused on following our plan of eating and physical recovery that we ... failed to delve into the issues that caused us to eat compulsively.*"

—*A Lifetime of Abstinence: One Day at a Time*, p. 9

Before OA I was an expert on the art of losing weight. I knew how to lose the weight and lose it quickly. Somehow, each time I lost weight, it always found its way back to me. In working a program of recovery in OA, the weight has had to come off much more slowly; I've experienced delayed gratification. In OA I have to allow time for my emotions and spiritual growth to catch up with the difference in body size. I need to earn my weight loss a day at a time and turn my ever-elusive goal weight over to the decision of my Higher Power. Through working an OA program, I am able to let go of the weight gracefully, and today, letting go of weight is a by-product of my spiritual growth. By maintaining conscious contact with a power greater than myself, I am finally able to feel at peace while abstaining from compulsive eating.

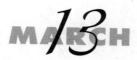

> *"We finally see there is a limit to how much we have been hurt. Our grievances are only so big and no bigger. The hurt had a beginning, and it can have an end as well."*
>
> —*The Twelve Steps and Twelve Traditions of Overeaters Anonymous*, 2nd ed., p. 61

In the silence of despair, my heart screams out for help. The weight of my sadness is too heavy to bear alone. Who can I turn to for help and understanding? Who will listen without judging me? Who will let me cry and not turn away from my tears? Who can I turn to when life seems unfair?

For years, I asked myself these questions. The hopelessness I felt was beyond measure. After coming to OA, I found answers that I had searched for all my life. I learned that I can turn to a Power greater than myself for help, a Power I call God. That Power is with me as I go for a walk, as I drive down a busy street, or as I sit quietly alone.

A sponsor understands my hurts, fears, and struggles with food. In meetings, I listen to people share about how they have used the Twelve Steps to work through their problems. OA literature gives me direction in working my program.

When faced with new hurts, I remember that this pain had a beginning, and it will have an end.

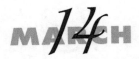

MARCH 14

"One aspect of this program that keeps us here is the promise of permanent recovery from this baffling disease."

— *The Twelve Steps and Twelve Traditions of Overeaters Anonymous*, 2nd ed., p. 69

Day after day I admit my powerlessness over food and everything else in my life. By turning my powerlessness over to God, I am accepting help. I ask my Higher Power to show me his will for me and for my ability to concentrate on recovery.

Reading Twelve Step literature reminds me that I have a disease and that I can recover, one day at a time. The program teaches me that I must commit to work and live the Steps. Maintaining abstinence, being accountable to my sponsor, giving service, and making amends are some of the actions that keep me in recovery. As I keep these commitments each day, I receive the healing, happiness, joy, and freedom that eluded me before program.

I am grateful to God, to my family, to my OA family, and to all who love me unconditionally for their part in helping me become the woman I am meant to be. Permanent recovery is possible, and I am worth receiving it.

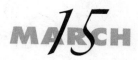

"For most of us, the central factor in this spiritual awakening has been our decision to trust a Higher Power with every aspect of our lives."

—*The Twelve Steps and Twelve Traditions of Overeaters Anonymous*, 2nd ed., pp. 81–82

The day I went to my first OA meeting in 1979, I was fat, miserable, and overeating continuously. At that meeting I received the gift of abstinence from compulsive overeating. I still ask for and gratefully receive the gift each day. This had to come from a Power greater than myself because I certainly did not cause this change.

Before OA I did not know God, and I did not recognize this spiritual awakening when I received it. I believe I received the gift of OA's Twelve Steps so I might recover from my disease. Applying those Steps to my daily living has changed my life, and the need to eat compulsively has left me.

Today I trust and depend on my Higher Power for everything in my life. Things always work out when I put them in God's hands.

To God: I love you, I trust you, and I thank you.

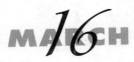

MARCH 16

"Some of us did not believe in God. We despaired of finding a solution to our problems if that meant we had to 'find God.'"

—*The Twelve Steps and Twelve Traditions of Overeaters Anonymous*, 2nd ed., p. 12

I specifically avoided coming into these rooms because I did not intend to deal with God. I came in simply because I wanted to gain control over my weight problem. I was an avowed agnostic; it was totally irrelevant to me whether or not God existed.

I had to "act as if" for several months. I did not realize that I had developed a real relationship with a Higher Power until I looked back on my OA experience and realized that my Higher Power had been the prime mover in my recovery all along. It was only when I became aware of all the gifts I had received that I asked who the giver was. What a shocking realization: because the gifts were surely divine, then, equally as surely, the giver must also have been divine.

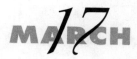

MARCH 17

"Because of our compulsive eating, we have turned ourselves into objects of ridicule and we have destroyed our health."

—*The Twelve Steps and Twelve Traditions of Overeaters Anonymous*, 2nd ed., p. 10

I was my compulsive overeating. I had lost my identity and all direction in my life. The insanity of trying to fill the emotional emptiness and the spiritual void with food consumed me. I lost my health, my ability to work, and my marriage to this disease. I am still without these, but I see the joy and freedom of recovery. I feel neither regret nor "if only," but simply a humble thankfulness that the craziness of my life managed to take the path that led me to God and to my daily recovery.

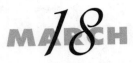

"The amazing secret to the success of this program is just that: weakness. It is weakness, not strength, that binds us to each other and to a Higher Power and somehow gives us an ability to do what we cannot do alone. We have discovered that if people in this program love us, it is not for our strength, but for our weakness and our willingness to share that with others."

—*Overeaters Anonymous*, 3rd ed., p. 4

How often have I been afraid to share with others my struggles or the return of the same old character defects—ashamed that I am not perfect and am not winning every round? Whenever I do find the courage to share, I find that people accept me much more readily than I ever accept myself. Program people share and applaud my victories, but it is their ability to accept my weaknesses that keeps me coming back.

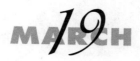

MARCH 19

"With practice, it becomes easier."

—*The Twelve Steps and Twelve Traditions of Overeaters Anonymous,* 2nd ed., p. 71

I'm a classical musician, and I know about the pain, discouragement, and boredom of practice. I make many mistakes, and I make them repeatedly. But a wonderful thing happens as I persist. As the mistakes fade away, the true beauty of the music emerges. I contact the soul of the music. It's a truly spiritual experience.

This OA program has been like that for me. Persistence has been the key. I've gone through periods of pain, discouragement, and boredom while practicing the program. I've heard people in the rooms say, "The only way out is through" and "Keep on keeping on."

With practice, my abstinence has become easier and cleaner. With practice, working the Steps has become easier and clearer. Things have become lighter and brighter with practice, the true beauty of my life has emerged, and I've contacted my soul.

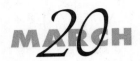
"As we complete Step Five, we may feel many emotions, among them humility, elation, and relief."

—The Twelve Steps and Twelve Traditions of Overeaters Anonymous, 2nd ed., p. 44

After I completed Step Five, many of my fears diminished, my attitudes changed, and my defects troubled me less. Simply sharing my defects with a trusted confidante caused these changes in me. I believed that the darker side of my emotions gave me little in common with others. After Step Five, I felt more a part of this world. For the first time, I could see the struggles of others and find compassion in my heart for them. We were not better or worse than each other. Didn't we all deserve the benefit of the doubt?

I had much work to do, but others had drawn the road map, and I became willing to ask for directions. Without the barrier of shame, my path didn't seem quite so desolate or lonely.

"God, grant me the willingness to see my imperfections as a means of getting closer to others and to you."

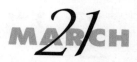

MARCH 21

"My life consists of single moments. I occupy them one at a time, savoring the fullness of each, and find there is no room for fear."

—*For Today*, p. 293

The joy of no fear. The joy of living and enjoying each moment as it comes. I am calm. I am worry-free and I don't have to jam too much of life into now. My moments are full but not overcrowded. I do one thing at a time. There is time in God's world to experience life. I am enough. I will do enough today to get the job done. There may not be any extra, but I don't need that. I am full.

Life is to be savored. Life is to be lived in small breaths, not huge gulps of air. Life can be tasted in small portions. God teaches me this, and he is my compass, my guide. I turn to him when I need a gentle reminder that he is in charge, and he has given us time today to do what we need to do to live happily, joyfully, freely whole.

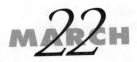

MARCH 22

"Getting out of my own way gives me the freedom to rise to the highest level of which I am capable."

—*For Today*, p. 280

I see the details and fret over them; my Higher Power sees the big picture. This is my Higher Power's plan for me:

To be free of fear;

To march after every single dream;

To recognize where my passion is;

To let my passion loose;

To be strong of mind, body, and spirit;

To grasp for all the good things that could be mine;

To love unreservedly;

To keep the real priorities in front of me;

To experience joy without limits.

When I am able to accept that this is my Higher Power's will for me, I see the need to stay out of the picture. My plan wasn't nearly as good.

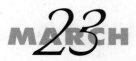

> *"We have eaten food that was frozen, burnt, stale, or even dangerously spoiled. We have eaten food off other people's plates, off the floor, and off the ground. We have dug food out of the garbage and eaten it."*
>
> —*The Twelve Steps and Twelve Traditions of Overeaters Anonymous*, 2nd ed., p. 9

The first time I read this passage I thought I had stumbled into some secret organization where someone was following me with a video camera. I thought back to the times I had hacked with a fork at some frozen dessert I had been saving for company. I thought about how my family nickname was "old garbage can" because I would finish whatever food anyone left on a plate. I had brushed the dog hair off fallen snacks (a little dirt won't hurt you) and poured dishwashing liquid on food in the garbage so I wouldn't fish it out. Suddenly I realized that my behaviors were common enough to appear in a book. I looked around the meeting and saw the faces of people with MY problem, and it was their problem too. For the first time, I could read the rest of the wonderful book and see myself in the answer instead of only in the problem.

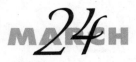

"At the very first meeting we attended, we learned that we were in the clutches of a dangerous illness, and that willpower, emotional health, and self-confidence, which some of us had once possessed, were no defense against it."

—*Overeaters Anonymous*, 3rd ed., p. 1

What a relief to discover that it wasn't just a matter of willpower! I came to OA in a state of demoralization. I just couldn't get a handle on diet and exercise. I'd quit drinking years before my first OA meeting, and quit smoking soon after I discovered I was pregnant. Surely I could muscle my way through this one. I understood about taking a leap of faith and surrendering my desire to drink to a Power greater than myself. I thought I should be able to handle food on my own. After all, it wasn't a drug. That's what I thought! OA taught me an entirely different perspective on food. I was an addict, and I was as addicted to diets as I was to junk foods. These things affected my mind, body, and spirit in the same way that alcohol had. I had to surrender to this obsession as well.

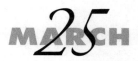

"Our heartfelt concept of God wasn't working."

> —*The Twelve Steps and Twelve Traditions of Overeaters
> Anonymous,* 2nd ed., p. 14

Years of praying, begging, and crying for release from this overwhelming need for more food have left me suspicious about the claims of Step Two. But I ask myself, what do I have to lose by thinking about this—a concept of God that hasn't worked for me? Could my ideas about God actually be preventing my recovery? This thought not only assaults the pride I have in my spiritual development, it also shakes the very foundation on which I've built my physical, emotional, and moral life.

As much as I recoil from such thoughts, a voice within me says that this notion may be an inspiration. Am I willing to free my spirit so I can envision a Higher Power that will indeed bring about recovery? Willingness is the beginning of the healing process, and today I will let my mind and spirit go beyond the limits of my experience, education, and emotions to find a Higher Power who is waiting to lead me to recovery.

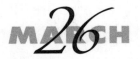
MARCH 26

"Never be in a hurry; do everything quietly and in a calm spirit. Do not lose your inward peace for anything whatsoever, even if your whole world seems upset. Commend all to God, and then lie still and be at rest in His bosom."

—St. Francis de Sales as quoted in *For Today*, p. 357

I calm down instantly upon reading that quote and the rest of that page. I give up control and know that my Higher Power will get everyone ready, in the car, and off to the appointment at the appropriate time. I realize that my job is to stay God-centered and loving, rather than bullying everyone.

This quote helps me even when I'm feeling calm. It always brings more peace to me and strengthens my bond with my Higher Power. God loves me and empowers me to heal more each day.

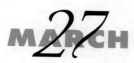

MARCH 27

"Before finding OA, I didn't know the meaning of the word 'balance,' and I didn't know that my life was unmanageable. I viewed the world in black-and-white extremes: Everything was either wonderful or awful, perfect or a total disaster."

—*Abstinence*, 2nd ed., p. 120

I have spent most of my life looking at myself and everyone else with a black-or-white check list. I allowed no gray areas, especially for myself. My greatest fear was that others would see my large black list and realize what a failure I was. This kept me from being close to others. I went out of my way to be friendly but ran from attachment and closeness because I feared the rejection that would surely follow.

In OA, I realize that I am not the only one who is imperfect. OA members, friends outside OA, and God—especially God—accept me as I am. In God, I have a loving and forgiving teacher who also guides me to the better way.

This has led me out of the black hole of fear and toward the bright white light. Thank you, OA!

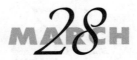
MARCH 28

"As we have dealt lovingly with every person in our lives, our spiritual awakening has become a reality."

—*The Twelve Steps and Twelve Traditions of Overeaters Anonymous*, 2nd ed., p. 67

One of the major results of working Step Nine is intimacy. Sometimes, because of the openness and vulnerability that are inherent in performing Step Nine work, I am communicating on a more intimate level with the person involved. At all times, because I am so grounded and open and willing to take risks, I am having conversations with my soul. I am more intimate with myself—that part of me that operates at a higher level, that part that coexists with my Higher Power.

Step work is entwined with the awareness of intimacy with my Higher Power, with others, with myself. Perhaps this is the reason the entire process is important, not simply the results.

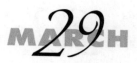

"Honesty is a key factor in our recovery from compulsive eating, and so we will want to develop this trait."

> —*The Twelve Steps and Twelve Traditions of Overeaters Anonymous*, 2nd ed., p. 44

It's one thing to be honest about what I did in the past or what I ate yesterday, but continuing this honesty in everything I do or say is another. I have found that as my growth in recovery continues, it becomes difficult for me to lie to myself, my Higher Power, my sponsor, or those in my circle of loving witnesses.

"The truth shall set you free" are words to live by. Maybe once I could lie about my weight on my driver's license or on some medical application, but today I do not hedge the truth.

Today, people can look at me and know that I am a person of my word. My integrity is important, and it comes from my truthfulness, harmlessness, and honesty.

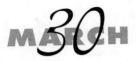

MARCH 30

"Service to our groups, service bodies, and OA as a whole has been a surprisingly powerful factor in our recovery."

—*The Twelve Steps and Twelve Traditions of Overeaters Anonymous,* 2nd ed., p. 83

When I first joined OA, I shied away from service opportunities. I told myself several things: "I'm too new," "I don't know enough about program to perform that particular service," "It will take too much time from my work or family," and, best of all, "In the past, I have given too much of myself and my time to other organizations. Since I don't know how to give in a healthy way, I'm going to be very cautious now."

In order for me to reap the benefits of service, I had to get over the hurdles I set up to sabotage my own attempts at recovery. I had to blindly volunteer to perform service even though I did not feel experienced enough or recovered enough or healthy enough to set appropriate limits around my service. Even though I thought I was making it easier for myself by not doing service, I was actually making it harder on myself by denying myself the Tool that so effectively enhances my recovery.

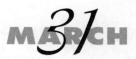

MARCH 31

"Have I been afraid to express myself, to tell others how I feel?"
—*The Twelve Steps and Twelve Traditions of Overeaters Anonymous*, 2nd ed., p. 31

I have an emotional and physical disease with a spiritual solution. Hiding my feelings from myself and others is certainly one of the roots of my illness. A Fourth Step can bring me into the light of day. But other Tools help shed that light as well. Every time I pick up the phone to call my sponsor or an OA friend, each time I take up my pen to write, I move myself along the path of freedom, awareness, acceptance, love, and recovery.

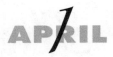

APRIL

"Made a searching and fearless moral inventory of ourselves."
—Step Four

This requires complete disclosure and absolute honesty. I can make no excuses for my behavior, only a bare-bones examination of my conduct. Action entails major Step work—working with a sponsor and processing the defects encountered. The ensuing grace is the result of living in the solution of the Steps and practicing each Step's spiritual Principles. This grace is abstinence and a reliance on my Higher Power. This grace is the new freedom promised to us all.

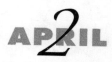

APRIL 2

"Repetition is the only form of permanence that nature can achieve."

—George Santayana as quoted in *For Today*, p. 204

This helps me remember that repetition in recovery is a wonderful gift, not the addiction to rote behavior that my relapse would have once had me believe. I felt angry that I had followed a food plan for over seven years, attended several meetings a week, kept eighty pounds off, and still relapsed. My new denial was not that I had a problem with food, but that the OA program would work for me. Though it worked for many others, I was convinced that it would not work again for me. And even if it would, it was only temporary—like everything else.

During my ten-year relapse, the repetition of the OA program sounded like an impossible chore. But today in recovery, I feel like OA's repetition has a beauty and a rhythm. It adds a life-saving structure to my day on three levels: physical, emotional, and spiritual. Conversely, the nightmare is repeated daily if I live in the disease. It can also achieve a form of permanence. So for today, I use the Tools and work the Steps to stay spiritually fit. And I accept that everyone's recovery, not just mine, is permanent only through repetition.

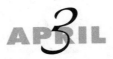

APRIL 3

"We were free to set aside theological arguments and examine the idea of spiritual power in light of our own desperate need for help with our lives."

—*The Twelve Steps and Twelve Traditions of Overeaters Anonymous*, 2nd ed., p. 13

Before OA, fear, anger, and sorrow filled my life away from the food, while I binged alone inside my house with a driven, trance-like numbness. Two things saved me: I recognized I desperately needed help with my life, and I believed OA would be the answer.

I channeled all my determination and self-will into working this program because I knew my life depended on it. I had to put aside all my agnostic theological arguments and act as if I believed in a Power that could help me.

My desperate need freed me to discover the energy source I now call God: the ultimate source of comfort, acceptance, love, and peace. God is the source of my abstinence and the source of my repose from the trials and tribulations of life on earth. I needed this disease to find this solution.

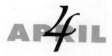

APRIL 4

"There is no finer way to treat people than to accept them as they are."

—*For Today*, p. 220

Truer words were never spoken. Lack of acceptance has been the cause of all our problems, according to the Alcoholics Anonymous Big Book. All my relationships changed the day I started accepting people exactly as they are. Occasionally I forget and revert to my old ways (critical, judgmental), but when I remember to control my instinctive reactions and feel compassion and acceptance for the person, rather than ridicule and rejection, I feel better. Other people are aware of my changed feelings and respond much better to me than they did in the past.

This is a powerful meditation for me. I remind myself daily to accept people exactly as they are, with all their frailties, shortcomings, and other human weaknesses. They are just like me: trying to get by in an often unfriendly world and poorly equipped to do so.

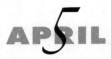

APRIL 5

"God is not my arms and legs. It is up to me to do the footwork. Ours is a program of action."

—*For Today*, p. 136

These words gave me a real wake-up call. I had been abstinent from compulsive eating for eighteen months and had seen some great improvements in my life. Many of the important relationships in my life had been healed and improved, many of the resentments I had carried for years were gone, I felt better about myself, and I had lost twenty pounds. But my weight was at a standstill. It was no longer enough to pray each day and say, "My Higher Power will take care of it." He did take care of it: He showed me those words. I must use my arms and legs and do the footwork. I must work the Steps, do my daily reading, writing, and praying. Most important of all, I must ask him each day to help me put down the food. It is my arms that put it in my mouth. I must ask for help from my Higher Power, my sponsor, and my group. That is where my strength and serenity come from, and that is how I will reach and maintain a healthy weight.

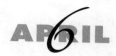
APRIL 6

"In Step Eleven, we are challenged to actively seek to improve our relationship with our Higher Power in the same way we might develop any relationship, by taking the time on a regular basis to be with HP."

—*The Twelve Steps and Twelve Traditions of Overeaters Anonymous*, 2nd ed., p. 76

Do I check in? When I am in a decision-making process or mode, do I run it by my Higher Power before taking action? Do I pray? Do I listen?

Using a mental alarm clock, I will set aside a specific time to check in with my Higher Power during my day. I got here (desperate, eating compulsively) by doing things on my own. I stay here (abstaining) by fostering relationships with my Higher Power and OA members.

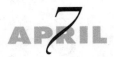

"The Tenth Step begins with the word 'continued,' our first clue that perseverance is about to become a key aspect of our recovery program."

—*The Twelve Steps and Twelve Traditions of Overeaters Anonymous*, 2nd ed., p. 70

I have persevered in this program through recovery, slips, and relapses. When someone asks why I go to meetings when I'm slipping and sliding, I say, "Because there is no other way." I have been mulishly stubborn many times in my life.

The OA program has taught me that stubbornness is about ego. I want it my way. I want to be in control. I've heard the acronym EGO for Easing God Out. When I live in EGO, I live in fear. My attempts to control are an attempt to wrap up my fears into a tidy parcel.

Perseverance, however, is about surrendering to my Higher Power. I've heard the acronym GOD for Good Orderly Direction. When I surrender, I am still responsible for the effort, but I leave the results to my Higher Power.

Stubbornness is ego-driven and fear-based. Perseverance is surrender to my Higher Power and is faith-based.

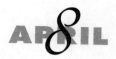

"We apply this Principle in many ways now, learning through each day's experience the difference between self-will and a simple willingness to cooperate with the guidance of our Higher Power."

—*The Twelve Steps and Twelve Traditions of Overeaters Anonymous,* 2nd ed., p. 85

Sometimes I have to remind myself that, "If I disagree with God, guess who's wrong?" By whatever means we were created, that creation process determines my eating needs. My health and well-being depend on my willingness to cooperate with that reality. I cannot do God's part; I never could, but as I operate in harmony with what God does, I am recovering.

It is the same with all of life's activities. Everything goes better as I cooperate with how things really work, by employing the Twelve Step Principles: honesty, hope, faith, courage, integrity, willingness, humility, self-discipline, love, perseverance, spiritual awareness, and service. When I started asking God to help me with his plans, instead of asking his help with my plans, I was on my way! Now I can welcome each new day because I am learning from my experiences.

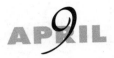

APRIL 9

"*Walking hand in hand with fellow OA members and our Higher Power, we are now exploring this world, using the great spiritual Principles embodied in the Twelve Steps as the map to guide our way.*"

— *The Twelve Steps and Twelve Traditions of Overeaters Anonymous*, 2nd ed., p. 86

What a wonderful way to think of our program: as a map to guide us as we live each day embodying the physical, emotional, and spiritual aspects of our lives. The Steps and Traditions are the path that takes us on this journey, outlining the elements as a cartographer would, illuminating and guiding our way.

From the First Step, in which I admit my powerlessness, to the Twelfth Step, in which I "practice these principles in all my affairs," I know what action I must take to continue my recovery. How nice to know that others are stepping the Steps and walking hand in hand with me. Above all, I know that a Higher Power is there beside all of us as we continue on the road of recovery.

For today, may I continue following the OA map as I step forward each day on the road of recovery.

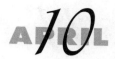

APRIL 10

"If we can share what we have learned, if we can apply it to all areas of our lives, we will have indeed performed the task for which we have been placed on this earth."

—*Beyond Our Wildest Dreams*, p. 122

This is the true essence of program: to continue sharing the OA message with all who share our compulsion. When we live the program and follow it in all our affairs, we set an example that shows others that OA works. It is more than talking about it; it is doing it.

The OA program has three A's: awareness, acceptance, and action. Our awareness begins at Step One and continues through the Steps, especially in Steps Four and Ten. Accepting our awareness comes gradually as we work the Steps. Then comes the action we need to take. For that we look to find God's will for us. Step Three is our starting point when we turn our lives and our will over to our Higher Power.

For today, by sharing what we have found and taking action in our lives, may we continue to carry OA's message.

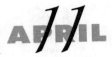

APRIL 11

"They want to learn all they can, and they never know whom their Higher Power might choose to teach them."

—*The Twelve Steps and Twelve Traditions of Overeaters Anonymous,* 2nd ed., p. 166

How often have I prayed to my Higher Power, asking for the solution to a problem or for deeper insight into my innermost self, yet ignored the answer when it was given. So many times I have sat in a meeting and discarded the useful suggestions of other members because they were still fat, were bulimic/anorexic, were of the opposite sex, or were too adamant. I had a multitude of reasons for ignoring others' ideas. If I am to reach a level of recovery that frees me to live a life of sane and happy usefulness, I must be willing to listen with an open mind and an open heart to all who share my compulsion. When I discard a suggestion because I find fault with the messenger, it is I who will suffer.

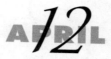

APRIL 12

"Practicing the Principle of faith today means that we no longer go through life acting however we feel like acting at any given moment. Instead, we look to our Higher Power for guidance and strength as we face each decision."

—*The Twelve Steps and Twelve Traditions of Overeaters Anonymous*, 2nd ed., p. 85

I used to sit on the fence, afraid of making decisions. What if I made the wrong decision? Faith in God has taught me that decisions need not scare me. As I work Step Three, I try to find God's will for me for each day. If I honestly seek his will, I believe I am practicing Step Three. I turn to God for guidance and wait for the intuitive knowledge that he provides. I have come to believe that there are no mistakes or "wrong" decisions—only different lessons. Whichever way I go, I learn something. I trust God to provide me with those lessons and look forward to learning and growing.

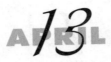

APRIL 13

"Humility, as we encounter it in our OA Fellowship, places us neither above nor below other people on some imagined ladder of worth. It places us exactly where we belong, on an equal footing with our fellow beings and in harmony with God."

—The Twelve Steps and Twelve Traditions of Overeaters Anonymous, 2nd ed., p. 52

I learned early on in life to measure myself against others, and being an obsessive person, I took this to an extreme. Thoughts such as, "Am I as pretty as she is? Am I as smart as she is?" constantly ran through my head. I saw myself as either inferior or superior to the person I measured myself against. The concept of being equal to others, yet still being unique and special, was a foreign concept to me until I attended a lot of OA meetings and worked the Steps.

Today I am working on valuing myself and others, just for who we are, without comparing or judging. When I am willing to listen to another person with compassion and an open mind, God shows me how valuable that person really is. And when I am able to honor another person's ideas and experiences, I am able to love and respect myself too, all in a spirit of humility and gratitude. Every person I encounter has something of value to contribute. Letting go of comparing and judging sets my spirit free.

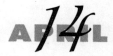

APRIL 14

"We gratefully follow in the footsteps of many others who have walked this way before us, and we're gratified to be making footprints of our own for others to follow."

—*The Twelve Steps and Twelve Traditions of Overeaters Anonymous*, 2nd ed., p. 86

I am grateful that all of you were here when I entered the doors of OA. I am grateful for the founders who left the first footprints for me to follow. I am grateful for the other compulsive overeaters who were willing and happy to share their experience, strength, and hope. I am grateful I didn't have to walk the path alone. Eventually, I found that I could leave footprints for others to follow. I, too, had experience, strength, and hope to share. I am always happy to share with others. We walk together on this path of recovery. We follow the footprints in the sand of those who have walked before us, and we leave footprints for those yet to come.

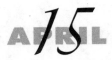

APRIL 15

"Sometimes, during the process of doing Steps Four and Five,
we become aware of more than our character defects. Sometimes
we uncover old traumas.... Until we began to deal with them,
some of us found that our abstinence was precarious or we
continued to feel unhappy, even while we were abstaining and
working the Steps."

—*The Twelve Steps and Twelve Traditions of Overeaters
Anonymous*, 2nd ed., p. 43

Why couldn't I stay abstinent? I had failed to tell another
human being my entire life story. I could not get abstinent, stay
abstinent, and live in recovery until I did so. I was the good
little girl who grew up to be the people pleaser. Paralyzing fear
seized my mind and body at the thought of telling someone
else what I had done. So I stayed in the disease. My humility
was born of greater trust in God and willingness to learn a
better way of living.

APRIL 16

> *"How do we get through these times without returning to compulsive eating? We don't panic. Instead, we quietly reaffirm our personal guidelines and ask our Higher Power to help us continue living within them. Then we turn away from food and eating to focus our attention on our OA Fellowship and the Twelve Steps."*
>
> —The Twelve Steps and Twelve Traditions of Overeaters Anonymous, 2nd ed., p. 21

I have to accept that the yearning for excess or dangerous food will return from time to time. But I can get through these trying times with my abstinence intact if I remember three simple words: Think, Pray, Act. First, I think about my abstinence, remembering the life of hell my sobriety has saved me from. I remember with gratitude what my abstinent life has given me. Then I reaffirm my plan of eating. Next, I talk to my Higher Power, asking for the willingness and ability to protect my most precious possession—my abstinence. Then I take action by picking up one of the Tools this program has given me and using it. If the compulsion remains, I repeat this process, using another Tool when I get to the action step. This three-part process works, without fail, if I work it.

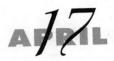
APRIL 17

"When we apply OA's Tradition Three, we find the treasure of friendship often where we least expect it, with people we once would have excluded from our lives. Such treasure is all around us, and all we have to do is open our hearts to receive it."

—*The Twelve Steps and Twelve Traditions of Overeaters Anonymous*, 2nd ed., pp. 111–112

After being in OA for a while, I look at who is in my life. The majority of my friends are those I met in these rooms, those who walk the path of recovery with me. When I think of my friends, sometimes I laugh. Most of them are not people who would have been my friends "in the real world." We seem to have little in common. The Big Book tells me that we are like those rescued from a sinking ship. We have in common the peril of compulsive overeating and the common solution found in the Twelve Steps. That provides a bond different from any I have experienced before. Many of these people I would have rejected as being too good for me or not good enough. I'm grateful that I saw the treasure of friendship and that God opened my heart to receive it.

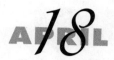
*"When we focus our discussions on the Principles embodied
in the Twelve Steps and Twelve Traditions, when we share
how we've found the solution to our eating problems through
practicing these Principles, we discover that we carry the
message to those who still suffer, and to ourselves as well.
No matter how much recovery we have, we still need to hear
the OA message."*

—*The Twelve Steps and Twelve Traditions of Overeaters
Anonymous*, 2nd ed., p. 120

As a group, our primary purpose is to carry "this message"
to those who still suffer. What is this message that I want to
carry? I want to carry the message of hope because that is what
others carried to me. When I came into OA, I had no hope.
Those who came before sometimes shared their problems and
always shared their solutions, found in the Steps, Traditions,
and Tools of our program. I often related to the problem and
always felt the hope in the solution. As I grew in the program,
I, too, had something to share. I often find that what I share in
a meeting is just what I need to hear. Yes, I do indeed carry the
message to myself. As I do, I remind myself of the hope found
in our common solution.

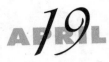

"As difficult as it is to shed old habits, I keep remembering the relief and freedom and joy that came the first time I tried abstaining one day at a time and not worrying about what would happen tomorrow."

—For Today, p. 293

I really wanted recovery from compulsive overeating. I attended meetings regularly, began working the Steps, and got a sponsor, but still the gift of abstinence eluded me.

I heard "one day at a time" repeatedly, but my suffering continued. Then one night my Higher Power spoke to me about "not worrying about what would happen tomorrow."

That was my first day of abstinence. God took my worry; I received his peace. Now I could understand what living one day at a time truly meant.

God, thank you for the gift of today. I am grateful for the freedom, relief, and joy I now feel.

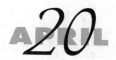
APRIL 20

"The 'compulsive overeater who still suffers' isn't always a newcomer to OA. She or he can also be an established member experiencing difficulties with the disease of compulsive eating or with other problems."

—*The Twelve Steps and Twelve Traditions of Overeaters Anonymous*, 2nd ed., p. 122

I was a compulsive overeater still suffering within OA. I struggled for ten years, trying to find the perfect abstinence and the perfect plan of eating. The doors of OA remained open to me, abstinent or not, and for that I am profoundly grateful. The Twelfth Step Within Committee formed at the World Service Business Conference says that we all have a place in OA and that our group's primary purpose is to carry the message. We carry the message not just to those who have not yet found OA, but to those of us in OA who are still suffering. Finally, the message reached me (or I reached for it), and I have abstained ever since.

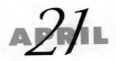
APRIL

"Sometimes we fail to be all that we could be, and sometimes we aren't there to give you all you need from us. Accept our imperfections, too. Love and help us in return. That is what we are in OA—imperfect but progressing. Let us rejoice together in our recovery."

—*Overeaters Anonymous*, 3rd ed., p. 5

Having been in OA a long time and having worked hard at OA's program for many years does not guarantee sainthood. I have often found these sentences helpful when I have needed to make amends for my failure to be available to a fellow sufferer.

Not only are these words a helpful approach to amends, they also help keep me in true humility. However long I have been in OA, I am a compulsive overeater. I am so grateful for my recovery that I will joyfully help when I can—but if I fail, then I will need help too.

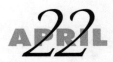
"Many of us find that the unconditional acceptance and trust that springs from the practice of anonymity opens us to one another in ways we have never experienced before."

— *The Twelve Steps and Twelve Traditions of Overeaters Anonymous,* 2nd ed., pp. 165–166

"How can I share things I've never shared before? I've never told anyone that." Those were my thoughts upon first learning about the Steps and Tools of this program. Anonymity answered my questions. It assured me that my sponsor or an OA friend would not repeat what I shared. I could trust, because trust is inherent in anonymity. When sharing my "deep, dark secrets," I experienced relief. I also experienced trust in another person and found that she trusted me as well. Because my sponsor shared some of her experiences, I knew that I was not alone or unique. She had to trust anonymity and trust me to share with me. That intimate sharing created friendships that last to this day. I can say anything to my trusted friend or my sponsor without fear. Their unconditional acceptance, love, and trust allow me to open up and recover.

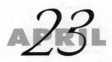

APRIL 23

"God loves us in our totality and is willing and able to help us in everything we do ... God will help us with every decision, even food choices and amounts."

—*The Twelve Steps and Twelve Traditions of Overeaters Anonymous*, 2nd ed., p. 14

Some of the most powerful tools in our "kit of spiritual tools" are the simplest. Our job is to open the toolbox and use one. Asking our Higher Power to feed us is one of those simple, yet powerful, tools that never fails us if we reach for it. I know that God would never hand me anything that would harm me or poison my life. Only the disease does that. Only the disease tells me that poison is a treat.

If I pause and ask before I make a decision about food or amounts, there will be a loving, peaceful space created in my day, and I will intuitively know what and how God would feed me if invited to do so. And when I listen and follow through with this sure guidance, that loving, peaceful feeling follows me throughout my day, and I know that I am loved, guided, and guarded always.

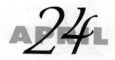

"Thus, it is to promote our own recovery that we cultivate the attitude of humility implied in Tradition Twelve. As we continue to grow spiritually, we begin to lose our desire for prestige in OA and in other areas of our lives."

—*The Twelve Steps and Twelve Traditions of Overeaters Anonymous*, 2nd ed., p. 167

I cultivate humility to promote my recovery. When I came into OA, I confused humility with humiliation. I had had enough humility in my life! I didn't need or want more. Over the years, I have learned that humility is different from humiliation. Humility means that I recognize I am not doing this alone. It means that I realize there is a God, and it isn't me! It means giving credit to the program, to the process of working the Twelve Steps and to my Higher Power, who is doing for me what I could never do alone. When I receive recognition in OA or in other areas of my life, I silently thank God, for I know that only through him have I achieved that for which I am being recognized.

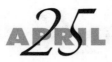
APRIL 25

"The most important thing in my life without exception is abstinence. I will do anything to keep it."

—*Overeaters Anonymous*, 3rd ed., p. 177

When I read this idea, I often bristle. Wait a minute, I think. God has put many roles in my life. I'm a wife, mother, sister, friend, employee. I have a home to run, family to coordinate, a job to manage. Surely, it is God's will for me that I use my energy, time, and talents to fulfill these obligations. If I put abstinence first, it could be at the expense of some other important activity. If I pray and meditate in the morning, my children will have to fix their own breakfasts. If I go to a noon meeting, I won't be able to run an office errand during my lunch break. If I take the time after work to call my sponsor and take calls from my sponsees, my husband may need to start dinner.

I have come to realize over my years in program that if I don't do these activities that support and maintain my abstinence, I may lose my abstinence. If that happens, I will become the pitiful, unattractive, unhappy person I was before coming to OA. My loving family and friends remember that person and willingly share tasks that free me to do those program activities that maintain my abstinence.

We all like the new me better than the old me. God bless them and me as I continue to make abstinence the most important thing in my life. Without abstinence, I have no life.

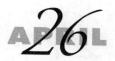
APRIL 26

"'What would I like such a Power to be and do in my life?' … Then we began to act as if such a Power existed, and we found good things happening to us as a result."

—*The Twelve Steps and Twelve Traditions of Overeaters Anonymous*, 2nd ed., p. 13

At first, the question reminds me of something mystical, like a child wanting his or her dream to come true. I believe that something magical does happen when I believe, trust, and act in faith that God will take care of me.

It is difficult for me to let go, wait, and "act as if." I want to look at things logically, and I need to see that two plus two equals four. I want it now, and I want it my way. It's very difficult for me to do the footwork, turn it over, and allow God to take care of the results. The times when I allow God to do this magic are when miraculous things begin to happen.

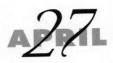

APRIL 27

"True comfort is to be found in the balance and sanity of abstinence. So deep and pure is this comfort that it is well worth whatever trouble or pain I might have to pass through to attain it."

—*For Today*, p. 253

Abstinence brings such peace and freedom to my life. It brings the simplicity of being able to wear anything in my closet, of not wanting to lie when I have to list my weight on my driver's license. The years of insomnia and nightmares are over because abstinence gives me the courage to be a person I respect and like and the integrity to align my actions with my values.

So when the seas of my life get stormy, I remember the phrase, "Abstinence is a lifeboat. Stay in the lifeboat." My disease used to tempt me into thinking being abstinent "made me" feel the pain. Today, I understand that the more uncomfortable my feelings, the greater the freedom I'll experience by walking through the situation abstinently. Now the time and energy I spent running is available for experiencing joy. For today, I treasure my abstinence.

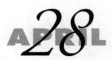
"We will no longer simply do what we feel like doing or what we think we can get away with. Instead, we will earnestly seek to learn God's will for us, then we will act accordingly."

> —*The Twelve Steps and Twelve Traditions of Overeaters Anonymous,* 2nd ed., p. 22

I sponsor in a very structured and precise way that has a spiritual Principle connected with each Step. Step Three is about commitment. Most compulsive overeaters find it difficult to keep their word. The first three Steps relate to building a foundation with God and to rebuilding our houses.

Commitment is crucial for the work that lies ahead in putting the house in order with Steps Four through Nine. What I once was able to eat or do before I took Step Three is no longer possible once I sign the contract with my Higher Power. Something happens when I have crossed the threshold and can no longer deny the truth about myself. I become real, honest, and true. In keeping that commitment, I have left the old self behind and must be willing to heed the voice of the new, recovering me.

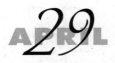

APRIL 29

"It is weakness, not strength, that binds us to each other and to a Higher Power and somehow gives us an ability to do what we cannot do alone."

—*Overeaters Anonymous*, 3rd ed., p. 4

Upset over the quality of my relationships, I was asked to examine defensive thoughts and actions that separated me from others. As long as I concentrated on the defects of other people, I was told, I would feel reluctant to ask for—and unworthy to receive—the help I needed. Sometime early in life, knowing that I lacked any effective defense against the urge to continually satisfy my selfish desires drove me shamefully inward. I fiercely protected that secret and learned to recognize that dark side in others like me. I sensed their awkwardness, and rather than identify myself as a kindred spirit, I exploited that knowledge in an attempt to feel superior. By alienating myself from fellow sufferers, my isolation guaranteed that the root causes of my addiction would go undetected, and they eventually overwhelmed me.

Today I know that I share a common problem. Through listening to others like me and giving of myself, I find my Higher Power and my recovery.

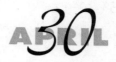

APRIL 30

"The amazing thing is that, as I grow in this program, I find less and less to be angry about."

—*For Today*, p. 90

Before OA I was angry all the time. Everything, including traffic, job challenges, fussy kids, or my uncooperative spouse would fill me with rage. My family never knew when I would explode. I consciously knew that the only way I thought I could calm down was to eat something sweet.

Then I found OA. Through my years of recovery I have learned to acknowledge and accept my anger, to work to figure out what caused it (either by talking or writing about it), and to get on with my life. Now this process often only takes seconds. I no longer even need to know why I am angry. I just am and I accept it. I don't want my body to be in that state, so I change my thoughts.

The most marvelous thing is that I find I am angry less and less. I accept that everything in my life is exactly as it is supposed to be. My Higher Power knows what is right. So what is there to get angry about?

MAY 1

*"Nothing in us can be changed until we first accept it.
Step Five, by helping us to know and accept ourselves,
makes it possible for us to change and recover."*

—*The Twelve Steps and Twelve Traditions of Overeaters
Anonymous*, 2nd ed., p. 41

Admitting the truth about myself requires honesty, the courage to tell the truth, and the willingness to accept it. Sometimes it seems like it is more than I can bear, but the only way to get it over with quickly is to go through it.

If I do not accept that I am sick, then I am not likely to seek any kind of medical treatment. If I am not willing to take my medicine, then it is unlikely that I will change and eventually get better. It comes down to how much I am willing to pay. If my time, money, and energy are not worth much, then I am not likely to pay the price. If living in recovery, enjoying life, and reaping the benefits are my primary concerns, then I am willing to pay the price and grow from that opportunity.

MAY 2

"What do we say when we talk with God? We say whatever we feel like saying."

—*The Twelve Steps and Twelve Traditions of Overeaters Anonymous*, 2nd ed., p. 77

What sets OA apart from the diets, clubs, and other programs for compulsive overeaters? A faith in a Higher Power that will restore me to sanity. And that Higher Power can be anything I choose it to be. I can choose God as I understand God, not as my parents understand God, or my community, my friends, or even my sponsor. It is my understanding that matters, no one else's. God comes to each of us in the way we can best understand. I need no formal ritual, no structured prayer to talk to my God today. I need only believe that God is with me, and God is here. I talk to God today as I do to my best friend. I seek guidance, ask for strength, and most of all, I say, "Thank you."

MAY 3

"Each group has but one primary purpose—to carry its message to the compulsive overeater who still suffers."

—Tradition Five

After ten years in OA, I had experienced a sixty-pound weight loss. But now I was in relapse—no meetings, no phone calls, no calls from others. Then one day two OA friends suggested that I bring drinks to Unity Day. I hesitated but said I would do it, hoping that I would forget over the next few weeks. But I didn't forget, and being "Miss Responsibility," I did what I said I would do.

At the meeting I didn't want to share, but a game led me to discuss the Fifth Tradition. I cried and shared about my relapse and the two friends who had called me and brought me back to OA. I have been abstinent, in recovery, and doing service ever since that day. I am most grateful to those two OA friends and encourage others not to forget the folks we haven't seen for awhile. We need them, and they may need us.

"All who have experienced the pain of compulsive eating and want to stop are equally welcome here."

—*The Twelve Steps and Twelve Traditions of Overeaters Anonymous*, 2nd ed., p. 108

When first introduced to the OA program, I was very weight-focused. I wanted more than anything to lose my excess weight as quickly as possible. I came to meetings sporadically and spoke to very few members. I would lose a few pounds and then leave the program for a while. Years later when I did become abstinent, I remembered how I felt during those times—I had no desire to refrain from compulsively eating. Instead, I wanted to diet. I did not take the suggestions seriously. Tradition Three illustrates the reason for my inability to grasp this program. I wanted the weight loss and even the pleasure of it without having to earn it first. Today when I watch newcomers struggle with the program as I did, I try to show the same compassion and acceptance as those before me.

MAY 5

"We learn to give our loving support to others freely, without trying to advise people or change them."

—*The Twelve Steps and Twelve Traditions of Overeaters Anonymous*, 2nd ed., p. 142

A woman said to me: "I will support you in a way that you have never been supported before." I did not understand what she was trying to say. I have confused support with action. I learned that the woman was saying: "I am behind you 100 percent and will support you in whatever you do. If you need something from me, then you have to ask for what you want."

This woman was allowing me the freedom to decide what I needed. She was not there to tell me what to do or even how to do it, unless I asked her to help me. Her approach was different from anything I had encountered before. It takes courage and willingness to receive such unconditional love and support.

MAY 6

> *"Abstinence means freedom from the bondage of compulsive overeating."*
>
> —*Overeaters Anonymous*, 3rd ed., p. 3

This statement is a profound revelation to me. It helps me remember when my disease wants me to forget that overeating dominated me for nearly four decades before I came to OA. Hearing these words early in recovery gave me a positive perspective when I felt deprived by abstinence or different from other people. Through ten years of abstinence, my appreciation of "freedom from bondage" has deepened physically, emotionally, and spiritually.

I cherish the precious independence OA has given me:

- Freedom to look in the mirror and like what I see.
- Freedom to purchase clothes I want, not just clothes that fit.
- Freedom to move my body in ways that morbid obesity prevented.
- Freedom to know all my feelings and to feel them fully.
- Freedom to become a life-managing adult.
- Freedom to connect with my loving Higher Power.

MAY 7

"Live and let live."

—program slogan

I was sitting at my sewing machine trying to get it to do a different stitch. The only stitch the sewing machine would do was the hemming stitch. I changed levers and pushed buttons, but the results were the same.

The thought then came to me. No matter how I try to change others, they have their own uniqueness. If they need to change, God will do the changing.

Showing love and respect for others as they make decisions in their life's journey leaves me free to make better choices in living my own life. My relationships will improve if I can love myself enough to let other people be responsible for their decisions.

"Live and let live" will free me from the compulsion to criticize, judge, condemn, and retaliate. Only then can I focus on the useful things in my life.

MAY 8

"At the very first meeting we attended, we learned that we were in the clutches of a dangerous illness, and that willpower, emotional health, and self-confidence, which some of us had once possessed, were no defense against it."

—*Overeaters Anonymous*, 3rd ed., p. 1

The only defense I have against the disease of compulsive overeating is a spiritual one. After years in the program, after weight loss, after learning and practicing healthy eating habits, after discovering better ways to react to life's changes, I must continue to search for and accept guidance from a Higher Power. How many times have I fallen for the mistaken notion that after a few days or months of successful eating and living, I can again take charge of my life? I've learned the hard way, by successive relapses and humiliations, that no matter how much better I look, act, or feel, God must always be in charge of my life. My continued recovery depends on the continual maintenance and growth of my spiritual condition. That hasn't changed from the day I set foot in my first Overeaters Anonymous meeting, and it never will.

"Honesty, hope, faith, courage, integrity, willingness, humility, self-discipline, love, perseverance, spiritual awareness, service, unity, trust, identity, autonomy, purpose, solidarity, responsibility, fellowship, structure, neutrality, anonymity, and spirituality: *These Principles, rather than our problems, should be the focus of every OA meeting.*"

> —*The Twelve Steps and Twelve Traditions of Overeaters Anonymous*, 2nd ed., pp. 120–121

Tradition Five says that "each group has but one primary purpose—to carry its message to the compulsive overeater who still suffers." I often wonder what "its message" is. This quotation clearly defines it for me. It is my responsibility to carry the message of the Twelve Steps and Twelve Traditions Principles. I can share my problems with my sponsor or a trusted friend. If I focus on at least one of the Principles, I ensure that I recover, that I share my recovery with newcomers, and that I contribute to the health and well-being of my group.

MAY 10

"Those of us who live this program don't simply carry the message; we are the message. Each day that we live well, we are well, and we embody the joy of recovery, which attracts others who want what we've found in OA. We're always happy to share our secret: the Twelve Steps of Overeaters Anonymous, which empower each of us to live well and be well, one day at a time."

—*The Twelve Steps and Twelve Traditions of Overeaters Anonymous*, 2nd ed., pp. 86–87

I have often told fellow OA members that if you really want to know how I work my program, you will have to follow me around for at least one day. Deception comes easily to this compulsive overeater. Through sheer force of my self-will run riot, I can appear to be working the perfect OA program. But to be the message, as this passage states, takes a commitment to working our Twelve Steps, to being abstinent, and most important, to sharing my successes, as well as my failures, with others. This commitment is one I must make continually, to live well and be well, one day at a time, with God's help.

MAY 11

"Looking back at how far we've come, many of us have been tempted to think we've arrived at the end of the journey."

—*The Twelve Steps and Twelve Traditions of Overeaters Anonymous*, 2nd ed., p. 82

Compulsive eating is an insidious disease. Many of the attitudes and beliefs we've clung to are also faulty and insidious. We always have to be on the lookout for them.

One of those attitudes is that we've finally arrived at recovery for good. Then we think we can slack off on taking all the actions that got us to this wonderful point in the first place: we don't attend as many meetings as we used to; we don't make as many phone calls or have a sponsor or give as much service as before; we may think we don't need to plan our food anymore or be as rigorously honest about it as we were; we may think that we don't need to keep studying and living the Twelve Steps and Twelve Traditions to the best of our ability.

We cannot rest on our laurels because in OA there are no laurels. There is only today, and only the actions we take for our program today determine how recovered we really are.

MAY 12

"Progress, not perfection."

—program slogan

I never thought of myself as a perfectionist; after all, I was overweight. How could I be a perfectionist? I've since learned that it has nothing to do with how you look. Perfectionism is a deadly character trait. It can kill as easily as compulsive eating. It taught me that I'd never measure up or get it right. And it was a lie. Progress, on the other hand, gives room to breathe, to be human, to make mistakes and get back on track anyway. Progress helps me become more flexible, accepting, and self-loving. Perfection feeds my dishonesty. Progress feeds my soul's desire for wholeness and health. I've come to believe that nothing in this world is perfect. Progress allows me freer choice and creates a healthy self-esteem. Perfection breeds disease and precludes self-esteem. I still experience my perfectionism, but because of OA and this slogan, I recover more quickly. I learn more from my mistakes than from trying to be perfect.

Today my program and my life reflect progress, not perfection. I see myself and my body as a work in progress. Today is good and I am blessed.

MAY 13

"*Tradition Five reminds us that our recovery doesn't come from simply discussing our problems with each other. It is in the OA message—in our Steps and Traditions—that we find solutions to our problems.*"

—The Twelve Steps and Twelve Traditions of Overeaters Anonymous, 2nd ed., p. 120

Before I found OA, I sought help from psychiatrists and a counselor. I became adept at talking about my problems. I was grateful for someone to listen to me describe my difficulties. But it was easy to slide into self-pity. I learned a lot about myself. I could analyze my past and came to see my past in a new way. I became better able to understand and love my mother. But none of these things stopped me from eating compulsively. It was only by attending meetings and working the program constantly that my compulsion was relieved.

"'Nothing tastes as good as abstinence feels.'"
　　　　　—*For Today*, p. 154

Before OA, I evaluated what I put into my mouth only by how good it looked and how good it would taste. I still catch myself yearning and reaching for yummy items. One of the best reminders for me is that "nothing tastes as good as abstinence feels." Years ago, before OA, a friend said this to me, but I never connected it to our program until I read it in my first year in OA.

Today, I know that immediate gratification is not the answer for me. Abstinence means exercise and sticking with the food plan that works for me. It gives me clarity, a sense of well-being, and the feeling that I am following God's will. Using the telephone and writing my feelings keeps me on track. Sponsoring is easier and more fun when I'm abstinent and working with my sponsor.

God, grant me the willingness to make healthy choices not only in the food I eat but also in my relationships, in my loving, and in my caring for others who are still suffering.

MAY 15

"... praying only for knowledge of His will for us and the power to carry that out."

—Step Eleven

"God, help me" was a simple prayer, a plea from a compulsive eater in relapse. Within an hour a person's name came to mind. I called her; she helped me on May 15, 1981. I have been abstinent ever since. I did not know that a simple prayer would begin my spiritual path. I turned to God with the food because I was desperate.

Today I am in love with God. He owns me. I trust him with everything. I experience the joy of his miracles in my life. I know the comfort of his consoling love when I am sorrowful. I watch his work in my life and in the lives of others. The God of my understanding is powerful and interested in everything about me. He guides and protects me, showing me the way. The Eleventh Step reveals the easiest and softest way: "... praying only for knowledge of His will for us and the power to carry that out." I trusted God with my food, and God has given me a life. That simple prayer, spoken long ago, still applies today, and God continues to answer me.

16

"One day at a time."

—program slogan

Taking each day as it comes makes my life so much simpler than it was before OA. It eliminates spending precious time looking back or looking ahead. Today is all I really have. Making each moment count is a big job. If, with my Higher Power's help, I do it well, there will be no time for idle projections or useless regrets.

That is not to say that I never need to look back or ahead, but that my day does not center on the past or the future. So much can be accomplished one moment, one hour, one day at a time. I try to tackle one task at a time, not sixteen like I used to. Taking this attitude gives me the freedom to tackle big or little problems, big or little jobs, big or little pleasures without getting all tangled up in "what-ifs" or "maybes" or "might-have-beens." One day at a time my life—spiritual, emotional, and physical—goes smoothly, no matter what is taking place.

"Once we compulsive eaters truly take the Third Step, we cannot fail to recover."

—*The Twelve Steps and Twelve Traditions of Overeaters Anonymous*, 2nd ed., p. 23

At one plateau in my recovery from the compulsive desire to overeat, I felt stuck—as if quicksand were sucking me down, smothering me in my compulsivity.

The difference between Steps Four and Five was confusing me. I didn't realize that Step Four was between my God and me and that Step Five represented my Higher Power's permission to let go in private confidence to a friend.

I had been spilling my Fourth Step for four months at OA meetings, but couldn't figure out why I felt stuck. I approached a sponsor with my dilemma. He granted me a private session in which he wisely tugged on an imaginary rope that would eventually guide me out of the self-made quicksand. He listened patiently, allowing me to ramble to exhaustion. Then his soft words tugged gently at the rope, telling me to take another look at my Third Step.

I left in a dither, eager to find another sponsor. I steamed for a week, until one day I picked up my OA *Twelve and Twelve* and started reading Step Three. When I read the line mentioned above, things clicked. I felt at peace. Those words became my promise. I began working on the Third Step again. Thanks to a wise sponsor and my Higher Power, my recovery resumed.

MAY 18

"Believe that you can be abstinent. You will be. Believe that you can have sanity, peace of mind and freedom to live the life you want. You will have them. Believe that you will recover. You will."

—*For Today*, p. 354

Believing in something that seems impossible requires a leap of faith. The gift of abstinence, freedom from compulsive overeating, the peace and sanity that result from working the program seem like elusive dreams to the newcomer or the relapser. Faith requires that I keep doing what works, no matter what. Sometimes it takes days, weeks, months, or even years before I can see and feel like I have gotten "it." And when I do "get it," I don't get to keep it because the "it" keeps changing.

The hope and belief that things will get better is not a tangible commodity that I buy; it is something I must earn. I believe it is possible for everyone to be abstinent, to recover, and to have all our dreams come true. We get what we expect, so "expect a miracle." We are all miracles.

MAY 19

*"Indecision is like the stepchild; if he doesn't wash his hands,
he is called 'dirty,' if he does, he is wasting the water."*

—Madagascan proverb as quoted in *For Today*, p. 247

This quotation and the paragraphs that follow it remind me
that I am not the only person who has problems with indecision.
I find strength in allowing myself to accept the reality of
human nature. Before joining Overeaters Anonymous, I had
to be perfect and instantly know the right answer to every
question. A lesson I fought hard against myself to learn is to
take a deep breath, relax, silently recite the Serenity Prayer,
and then decide. I still have to make decisions every moment.
Some I think through, some I don't, and some create anxiety.
The difference is that I'm not alone anymore.

MAY 20

> *"I continued to eat to soothe myself. Food comforted me when my parents did not."*
>
> —*Overeaters Anonymous*, 3rd ed., pp. 171–172

I feel sad when I think back to my days before OA—days filled with unstoppable eating, self-loathing, and anger. I felt alone in my world and kept myself apart from family and friends. Excess food sedated me, but it was never enough. I would swear not to binge the next day, but I couldn't stop eating.

After twenty-two years of coming back to OA, I now love myself first, which means I can love others. I started with OA members. They didn't reject me because of my size or eating habits. I rely on a Higher Power who loves me and allows me to accept myself as I am. I have learned to love myself, and therefore I can love others. I give service to others in and out of the program. I am alone, but lonely no more.

_"We responded to the love we had been shown in OA, by taking
action and working the Steps. The result was a new faith in
ourselves, in others, and in the power of that love."_

—The Twelve Steps and Twelve Traditions of Overeaters
Anonymous, 2nd ed., p. 15

Many OA people loved me until I learned to love myself.
It was not until I could love myself that I recovered and did
the needed work: used the Tools, worked the Steps, lived the
Traditions. It has been a long journey, but I have made it to
the other side: I am happy, joyous, and free.

"We were never meant to face this disease in isolation."

—*The Twelve Steps and Twelve Traditions of Overeaters Anonymous*, 2nd ed., p. 14

Before coming to OA, I had years of experience trying to find the diet, program, or motivation that would help me achieve and maintain a normal weight. Everything I tried led me to the same place, back to the overeating, the sickness, and the shame. What a relief it was to come to OA and plug into a support system of fellow compulsive overeaters. What a relief it was to say, "I'm powerless to stop eating compulsively," and to find people who understood. Not only did they understand, but they had overcome the same dilemma and willingly showed me the way. My isolation ended then.

Occasionally, I try to reclaim my isolation. I do it by being the know-it-all at OA meetings, by not really being honest with my sponsor, by being too proud to ask for help. Kept up long enough, this emotional isolation will land me back in that same place as all those pre-OA diets. Getting to meetings, doing service and calling my sponsor are not enough to keep me abstinent today. I must be willing to ask for help. That's the only way I can practice the Principle of humility in all my affairs.

"Clearly, if we are to live free of the bondage of compulsive eating, we must abstain from all foods and eating behaviors that cause us to eat compulsively."

    —*The Twelve Steps and Twelve Traditions of Overeaters Anonymous*, 2nd ed., p. 4

I like the simple approach of three meals a day, with nothing in between. My spiritual and emotional recovery can start from there. I don't need to punish myself with excess food. Working the program of recovery on all three levels, I have learned to love myself enough to want recovery and be willing to do the footwork required to get and retain abstinence.

"In Step Three, we learned faith as we made the most important decision we had ever made, the decision to trust God—as we understand God—with our will and our lives."

—*The Twelve Steps and Twelve Traditions of Overeaters Anonymous,* 2nd ed., p. 85

For many years, Step Three to me was nothing more than a decision to be willing. The Principle of faith was the key I had been missing. This reminds me of the parable, "If only I have faith the size of a mustard seed—miracles can happen."

When I applied the God Power I found in Step Two to the decision I made in Step Three, I found the willingness to carry on with the rest of the Twelve Steps and to remain abstinent from compulsive eating. It was then I allowed the miracles to begin.

MAY 25

"This abstinent way of life continues on a daily basis so long as we continue to trust a Higher Power with our lives, renew our Step Three commitment daily, and practice all of OA's Twelve Steps."

—*The Twelve Steps and Twelve Traditions of Overeaters Anonymous*, 2nd ed., pp. 21–22

As the holiday seasons approach, sometimes my disease wants to convince me that I can take a break from the discipline of my commitment to this program. That is when I need to remember that I still have some "fat in my head." Recovery is a one-day-at-a-time procedure that requires time for clearing away the debris of the past. I can do this best by adding more meditation, more meetings, and more service, rather than by taking time off.

"Abstinence is a new life, not in theory but in practice. It means following suggestions, listening to someone who knows more than I do about living abstinently."

—For Today, p. 203

The old me always knew the answers, always had the good ideas, never listened or followed anyone's suggestions. It was self-will running riot. Now, when I read something in OA literature, hear something at a meeting, or my sponsor shares something with me, I take it to heart and search for a place to fit it into my life. I reflect on how I can make it work for me, how I can adapt it.

With this disease of compulsive overeating, I cannot afford to be selective. Whatever is presented to me is presented for a reason, and my job is to absorb it. My OA recovery cannot be stagnant, nor can my progress be put on hold. I cannot control this progressive disease of compulsive eating.

Keeping myself open to other overeaters' perspectives and to God's will keeps me alive. Thank you, God, for the insight and experiences shared by others. The circle of life for me is Step work and abstinence from compulsive overeating. I apply what I hear to my daily routine, thus becoming and staying spiritually sound, emotionally secure, and physically fit.

"Just staying abstinent—if it's all I can do today—is reaching for recovery."

—*For Today*, p. 167

Only from repeated failures have I learned that I must have spiritual fitness to have abstinence. These two are intertwined like the chicken and the egg. I can't have one without the other. When I notice any negativity forming within me, I pause to see what's going on; then I take some positive action, even if it's only to rest.

Whenever I have a craving or feel an impulse that could lead me away from my abstinent lifestyle, I gently say no to myself, like a mother leading her toddler away from danger. This mother did not raise me. OA planted the seed of this mother in my heart. Only I can take that first step away from the food and toward my Higher Power and the Tools of Recovery, slogging through those moments, hours, or even days of craving and negativity. I point myself away from them, toward the Tools and God's love.

"We seek to examine our actions, in particular to identify where we were resentful, dishonest, fearful, self-seeking, and inconsiderate, so we can learn from our mistakes and build on our successes."

—The Twelve Steps and Twelve Traditions of Overeaters Anonymous, 2nd ed., p. 72

Do I take a thorough look—an inventory of my conduct—when I do a Tenth Step? Or do I focus more on my feelings and thoughts? There's a world of difference between self-examination and self-awareness. The first means scrutiny of my behavior; the second relates more to my state of being. For me to be successful with the three-fold process of self-examination, meditation, and prayer as described in Steps Ten and Eleven, I need to scrutinize my conduct. I ask myself where in my day I could have been more honest, willing, self-disciplined, and loving. How can I apply these Principles to my daily life? Usually by more meditation, more prayer, more practice. Show me the way, Higher Power. Your will be done, not mine.

"When the individual accepts, on an unconscious level, the reality of not being able to handle compulsive overeating, there is no residual battle."

—*Overeaters Anonymous*, 3rd ed., p. 202

I have found this to be true. When I totally accept Step One, my compliance with the program and my abstinence are easy. The difficulty is that it is not easy to accept such total powerlessness. A corner of my mind will start to fear the utter helplessness and resist. Then there is a battle in my own mind. The battle opens up a breach through which the disease may enter.

I have found it useful to have a standard of total acceptance at an unconscious level, and I compare my acceptance of Step One with this standard. I know I cannot walk through a brick wall, and I've totally accepted this fact, so I don't try. I don't even resent the fact that I can't do it. When I accept Step One as completely as this, I am easily abstinent. I am free.

MAY 30

"When working this Step, we do more than just recite thoughts, words, and actions from the past that we consider to be our wrongs.... We need to look at what those actions have cost us."

—The Twelve Steps and Twelve Traditions of Overeaters Anonymous, 2nd ed., p. 42

It is very difficult for me, in doing a Fifth Step, to discuss the payoffs as well as the costs of my character defects. It helps to admit to an outside source that there were rewards, however small, in doing much of what I did. In reviewing the rewards, however, I can see how small they were compared to the costs today. I get to hear myself acknowledge that the payoffs are no longer worth the pain. When I hear myself saying this out loud, I know I have come a long way toward accepting it as my truth.

MAY 31

"Those who have studied them carefully have found that these Traditions can be applied effectively to all human relationships, both inside and outside OA."

—The Twelve Steps and Twelve Traditions of Overeaters Anonymous, 2nd ed., p. 89

I am grateful to the Traditions that keep our groups and OA as a whole functioning in a healthy way. I am also grateful that I can apply these Principles to all my relationships, whether anyone else knows about the Traditions or not. It's amazing how these simple ideas can improve my interactions with others. For example, what relationship can't be made better if I consider our common welfare and strive for unity? I can place God as the ultimate authority over all my relationships and pray to be a trusted servant, instead of a controller. I can allow others to be autonomous, unless a matter affects our relationship as a whole. Remembering to place principles before personalities helps me in all my relationships and dealings with other people. It is such a relief to simply look at the issue at hand and not get caught up in the personalities involved.

JUNE

"Were entirely ready to have God remove all these defects of character."

—Step Six

I recognize many of my character defects when I react strongly to seeing them displayed by other people. When I notice character defects in others and realize that I still practice them myself, even though I don't want to, I know I need God's embrace. For me, the first stage of Step Six is to accept that I have weaknesses and to know that God embraces me nonetheless.

JUNE 2

"Before I turn a problem over to God, I am reasonably sure that God expects me to take a stab at doing my part."

—*For Today*, p. 179

Before coming to OA, I spent my whole life expecting God and other people to solve my problems. I never tried to do what I could—my part. This quote helps remind me that there are things I can do to help myself. It helps me to have confidence in my ability to take care of myself. It shows me that I am responsible for my feelings and actions. God is gentle, but firm, in wanting me to do all I can for myself first. I couldn't handle food on my own, but I had to get to OA before God would help me with the food and my unmanageable life. What more could I ask for? I now have a loving Higher Power and friends to support me. I feel immensely grateful.

JUNE 3

"Any action, no matter how small, can help us overcome procrastination."

—*The Twelve Steps and Twelve Traditions of Overeaters Anonymous*, 2nd ed., p. 27

One thing I keep learning in various ways is how differently I can feel after taking one small action to change my circumstances. Usually, when I am frozen and immobilized by fear, I think of a hundred things I need to do, should do, or have to do. Yet I do nothing and hate myself more. Often someone else gently reminds me that I only need to do one thing to break the cycle. I don't need to jog five miles; a short walk around the block is a start to clearer thinking. The house doesn't need to be spotless, but making the bed makes my life feel more manageable. I might not be able to adhere to that "perfect" food plan, but am I willing to stop eating right now? It is the long view that overwhelms me. If I remember to pray for the willingness to do one small thing, I am living evidence that mountains can be moved by the results. I pray to be willing to do something for my recovery today. I pray to let go of the results and be willing to take the action.

"We are powerless over each of our defects of character, just as we are powerless over the food. Our character defects need to be removed by a Power greater than ourselves; we cannot do it alone."

—The Twelve Steps and Twelve Traditions of Overeaters Anonymous, 2nd ed., p. 47

For the longest time, I thought it was up to me to make my character defects go away, to try hard to be a better person, to battle knee-jerk reactions and force a new personality to emerge.

I came to see that the process was much more gentle. I'd already seen the benefits of letting my Higher Power work on my food problem. The awkwardness I felt about my imperfections became a catalyst to move ever closer to my Higher Power.

By acknowledging my powerlessness and asking for help in my prayers, I received new insights, much needed self-restraint, and the ability to negotiate stormy waters without leaving a wake of disturbance in my path. My program became a living mechanism to guide me toward becoming a kinder, more approachable human being and allowed me to prepare for reckoning with the wreckage of my past.

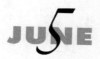

JUNE 5

"Each day that we live well, we are well ... one day at a time."
—*The Twelve Steps and Twelve Traditions of Overeaters Anonymous*, 2nd ed., p. 87

Today I can plan my recovery and follow that plan to the best of my ability. I do the things that help me live well: being abstinent, exercising, meditating, writing, and maintaining social contact. I concentrate on what I can do, not on what I cannot do. With God's help, I can live the message of the OA program, one day at a time.

JUNE 6

> *"We then find that, to deal with our inner turmoil, we have to have a new way of thinking, of acting on life rather than reacting to it."*
>
> —*Overeaters Anonymous*, 3rd ed., p. 2

It seems that all my life had been a series of reactions, either from fear, anger, or resentment toward others or situations, or from my own negativity or shame. To deal with my despair and inner turmoil I had to stop blaming life and find a new way of thinking.

With help from the OA program and my Higher Power, I learned that I can accept others as they are. I learned that I am not a victim of life. I can care for and be responsible for myself and my thinking. I can consciously choose positive thoughts and decisions that enable me to act on life one day at a time.

Any time that my food obsession returns, it is a sign for me that I need to look at my reactions to people and things. I need to willingly take responsibility for my part, and for my happiness. I need to own my own power to take action.

Today I follow the Twelve Steps and act on life.

JUNE 7

"It is the great paradox of the Twelve Step program of Overeaters Anonymous that we make a commitment to sane eating for only twenty-four hours in order to achieve a lifetime of recovery from compulsive eating and compulsive food behaviors."

—*A Lifetime of Abstinence: One Day at a Time*, p. 1

These words remind me that abstinence requires commitment and consistency. Commitment means I put abstinence first—before anything or anyone. This may sound selfish, but staying abstinent is the only way I can take my focus off food and put it on others. Commitment means I plan ahead for the right foods at the right times and do the spiritual work that allows me to access my Higher Power. Consistency means I recommit to abstinence each day—no excuses. These words remind me that I am not a victim of a disease about which I can do nothing. I alone am responsible for accessing the Higher Power that keeps me abstinent.

JUNE 8

"... praying only for knowledge of His will for us and the power to carry that out."
—Step Eleven

This last part of Step Eleven has become my natural response to the problems in my life, especially those that involve another person. I clung to it as a prayer during one of the worst times of my life. The quicksand of denial had caught me, and I was enabling my son to stay on drugs. In my confusion and pain, I turned to these words for the guidance and strength to do the right thing. I typed this prayer and kept it with me to remind me of what action to take when I wanted to run.

As I consciously contacted God through this prayer, my mind would clear and let me focus on God's will. Peace came when I knew he would give my son and me the power we needed to do his will. This simple prayer was a way I could touch God and pray for my son and myself at the same time.

"I have been given back the choice to eat compulsively or not, and I fully understand what I stand to lose if I fail to acknowledge this gift each day."

—*Overeaters Anonymous*, 3rd ed., p. 150

Often when I am in eating situations, I begin to hear excuses that start out, "I shouldn't, but ..." These days, I certainly do not have to play into others making excuses for their eating. Good planning and checking in with my sponsor means I don't have to avoid such occasions. I often take my planned food with me and do "my thing" while they do theirs. If it isn't time for me to eat, I can be content; I know that what I do keeps me on an even keel, and that is precious to me.

I used to make excuses, too, but I nearly went crazy with schemes to make up for it later. By practicing gratitude in my daily writing, I find I have several good ways to complete the sentence, "I'm glad to eat the way I do now, because ..."

JUNE

"When we face the guilt that truthfully tells us, 'You made a mistake,' we're freed of shame that falsely tells us, 'You are a mistake.'"

—*The Twelve Steps and Twelve Traditions of Overeaters Anonymous,* 2nd ed., p. 36

This quote helped me finish my inventory. Once I had shared the mistakes I've made with another human being and was helped to see my assets, I was amazed that my life went on. With the help of the program, the Fellowship of Overeaters Anonymous, and my Higher Power, the feeling deep within that the core of my being was rotten has left me. A day at a time, the need to destroy myself with food is taken away from me as I face the scars of my disease.

JUNE 11

"I have to be careful about my attitude toward anger."
—*For Today*, p. 90

Righteous anger is the hardest for me to release. I get such a good, self-affirming feeling from holding on to it. However, anger, like fear, takes up so many mental megabytes that there isn't room for new information and new feelings, new insights and new paths to conversation with my Higher Power. If I allow my hard drive (my heart) to fill to capacity with anger or fear, then there is no room for the positive, for what my Higher Power wants for me in life.

When the anger or the fear is gone, what's left? At one time I speculated that nothing would be left of me once I shouted or cried it all out and released it. Now I realize that what happened was a massive blackboard erasure with a whole new background—life—to fill as I want.

JUNE 12

"What we are entirely ready for, actually, is to have the difficulties our defects have caused us removed while we hang on to the defects themselves."

— *The Twelve Steps and Twelve Traditions of Overeaters Anonymous*, 2nd ed., p. 46

I took a moral inventory in Step Four, told it to someone in Step Five and was ready to proceed. Why did Step Six seem difficult? I had identified the character defects that caused me trouble, and they didn't appear to be things that anyone would want to keep. Resentments, angers, and fears ran my life. Writing them down had shown me how useless they were. I couldn't understand why I would still rant and rave or be fearful or jealous. I thought I wanted the defects removed. Maybe I wasn't trying hard enough. This sentence gave me the answer. I wanted to yell at my son, but I didn't want him to yell back or act angry. I wanted to make sarcastic comments, but I didn't want to hurt anyone's feelings. I wasn't willing to have my defects removed; I was just willing not to suffer the consequences. This sentence showed me that I had much work to do.

JUNE 13

"Sacred Awe!"

> —Nikos Kazantzakis as quoted in *For Today*, p. 342

I found this phrase so many years ago when I first started program. It has become such an important part of my program, for it helps to explain the unexplainable.

I am filled with Sacred Awe over the many riches and experiences this program has given me:

- the many "just for today" days of abstinence—this I will never be able to explain!
- the emergence and growth, through studying the OA Twelve Steps and Twelve Traditions, of many wondrous relationships.
- a loving Higher Power. He is always there for me, if I'm willing to ask.
- the many caring people within program that make it a Fellowship.
- the budding relationship with the lovely person whom I like: ME!
- the new, renewed, or increased awareness—the peace—the hope that I see and feel—the recovery that I am offered— the opportunity to try again today—hearing another's story of strength and hope—all the wonderful gifts I've been given.

Never, ever am I able to explain any of this, so I am continually filled with Sacred Awe. This is a God-given program, and my Higher Power has chosen me to experience—to live in—Sacred Awe!

JUNE 14

"Giving up control means growing up: my experience broadens, my pleasures expand, my usefulness to others increases and my horizon—like God's world—is limitless."

—*For Today*, p. 234

I used to believe that there were only three ways of doing something: the right way, the wrong way, and my way.

My expectation of others was that if they did it my way, we wouldn't be having these problems. I once operated under this belief and tried to control people and situations.

Today I realize that each person perceives the world with blinders on and filters out information that is contrary to his or her belief system. When I move the tiniest bit to the left or the right, I alter my view of the world, and I change my attitude.

The possibilities are limitless. One hundred people can view a situation in one hundred different ways, and all of them can be right. Today I am open to the possibility that God's world and his children have no limits.

JUNE 15

"*This miracle of sanity, the result of working OA's Twelve Steps, is an everyday reality for thousands of recovering compulsive overeaters.... It is possible for us to continue eating moderate, nutritious meals, one day at a time, day after day, month after month, year after year.*"

—*The Twelve Steps and Twelve Traditions of Overeaters Anonymous*, 2nd ed., p. 21

Yes—there is hope and a promise for me too! I am not a rudderless ship left unsupported to be tossed about upon an angry sea. I can find my way out of this agonizing existence and reclaim my tortured soul. The stark truth is no less than this: to get out of the hell of compulsive overeating, I must be willing to give up compulsive overeating, one day at a time. Simple, but not easy. A plan of eating helps keep me honest. I pray for willingness until it comes. I reach out to others to receive help and strength, and to give away what I have received. Most importantly, I work the Steps to the best of my ability. And in doing so, I reconnect with my Higher Power and find my way home to sanity and peace of mind.

JUNE 16

"We will no longer simply do what we feel like doing or what we think we can get away with."

—*The Twelve Steps and Twelve Traditions of Overeaters Anonymous*, 2nd ed., p. 22

This translates into one word for me: discipline, a word that my disease hates. I like the results I get from discipline, but I don't like the pain, discomfort, and patience it requires. That's where I must trust a Power greater than myself. By trusting my Higher Power and desiring to do his will, I'll want to do the next right thing and even know what the next right thing is. I get the "wants" by going to OA meetings, praying, writing, following a food plan, and exercising. All these things are good for me, and I do them despite my disease screaming in rebellion. No longer can I just do the things I can get away with or that I want to do. I am working an honest program while I learn to live with integrity and hold my head high. Slowly my will is changing and aligning with my Higher Power's will, one day at a time. It works if we work it. Don't leave before the miracle happens—the miracle of recovery from compulsive overeating. It happens!

JUNE 17

> "At one time or another, since we joined OA, most of us have experienced a period of complete freedom from the obsession with food and the compulsion to overeat."
>
> —*The Twelve Steps and Twelve Traditions of Overeaters Anonymous*, 2nd ed., p. 18

When I came into OA, I lost my weight swiftly by eliminating the foods I binged on. Later I learned that I was allergic to these foods. I began to analyze which was worse: the compulsion to overeat, or the obsession with food. I finally knew it didn't matter. I am a compulsive overeater, and that entails both the obsession and compulsion. I overcame both by working the Steps. The compulsion to overeat left first because I gave up my binge foods. After some time, the obsession with food itself, and all the games I played with food, also left. This way of life has given me such a gift!

I feel free now to live the life my Higher Power always had ready for me. For a long time, I chose food to cover up many things: fear, shame, guilt, anger—but also joy, happiness, serenity, and contentment. Now I live by these Twelve Steps. Without this daily contact, I would be back into the food, and I would surely die.

JUNE 18

"We can confidently face any situation life brings because we no longer have to face it alone. We have what we need any time we are willing to let go of self-will and humbly ask for help."

—*The Twelve Steps and Twelve Traditions of Overeaters Anonymous*, 2nd ed., p. 23

We entered OA knowing we had a problem with food, but we may not have realized the extent to which we had problems handling life. Using the Tools and listening to our sponsor and others at meetings can help us know what changes we need to make. Working the Steps also helps us to see how fear, control, self-pity, and self-centeredness enter into our daily lives. Steps Three and Eleven teach us to turn over the events of the day, ever reminding us that we do not have to face any day alone. This program works when we aren't navigating by ourselves. Our Higher Power and others will be here today to help us if we let them. The future may seem frightening; the past may have held pain, but today can offer us wonderful gifts we have yet to imagine. I can let go and let my Higher Power help me through this day.

JUNE 19

"I look at my past in order to understand myself and in order to let the past go."

—*For Today*, p. 235

As a compulsive overeater, I tend to be an all-or-nothing kind of person. I have found it best to simplify my life, eliminating as much clutter as possible. My life is a constant recycling process. However, in the case of relationships and past experiences, it's impossible to erase or ignore those feelings and memories.

I also tend to want to run or go for the quick fix. By practicing the spiritual Principles of the program and utilizing the Tools of Recovery, I confront my demons and work through my greatest fears. The process of uncovering, discovering, and discarding is an ongoing adventure. Detaching myself from what I believe happened, accepting what is true, and staying in the present moment serve to remind me that only this moment matters. Experience is what happens to me, but what matters most is what I do with that experience.

"There may be times when we're faced with an important decision and want to know our Higher Power's will. Our sponsors or OA friends might suggest that we pray about it, asking God to increase our desire to take the action if we are supposed to take it, or decrease our desire if we're not supposed to take it."

— *The Twelve Steps and Twelve Traditions of Overeaters Anonymous*, 2nd ed., p. 80

I believed that if I willed something strongly enough, then life would be perfect. Bingeing on food helped me maintain the illusion that I was in control. Eventually, the pain of eating became more unbearable than facing reality. The unconditional love from my Higher Power and OA gave me the courage to accept the truth and change.

I still feel confused sometimes when I have a decision to make. I try to meditate and ask God for guidance. Asking God to increase or decrease a desire was a breakthrough in my way of praying. I used to tell God what I wanted. Today, I try to pray for what I need and trust that God will take care of the rest.

JUNE 21

"Working the Steps will help us to let go of fear and indecision. If we are sincere, our Higher Power will give us the knowledge of our best course in life."

—*The Twelve Steps and Twelve Traditions of Overeaters Anonymous*, 2nd ed., p. 22

I realize that my Higher Power is giving me guidelines when …

I think of a course of action or a solution that is entirely new or different for me. This way I know the idea wasn't mine.

I see other people struggling with similar problems, and I recognize how the OA solutions have worked for them. This is God's way of showing me, by example, what works.

I realize that an unplanned event or person has literally popped up in my life. Then I know it's a "God thing."

JUNE 22

"The truth, learned from the experiences of thousands of OA members, is that, no matter how great our physical, emotional, and spiritual transformation, we still aren't cured. This is true even when we've reached the goal of a healthy body weight, even when we've worked all Twelve Steps to the best of our ability, even when we've celebrated milestone anniversaries of abstinence and recovery, even when we've been placed in positions of trust by other OA members and have rendered service to our groups and service bodies."

—The Twelve Steps and Twelve Traditions of Overeaters Anonymous, 2nd ed., p. 82

Unlike other groups or organizations we've been a part of, there is no "graduation" in OA. Another word for graduation, however, is "commencement." With OA, we commence a new life. This goes beyond the food and carries into all aspects of our lives, permeating our very beings. I no longer have to depend upon a calendar or graph to chart my progress. I work the Twelve Steps daily in a never-ending cycle. By doing this, I'm off the merry-go-round of dieting and into sanity and happiness. I'm thankful to OA for the endless beginning of my life.

JUNE 23

"We express our desire to become more effective in serving and helping others as our shortcomings are transformed into assets."

—*The Twelve Steps and Twelve Traditions of Overeaters Anonymous*, 2nd ed., p. 54

I read Step Seven many times but missed this part: my shortcomings will be transformed into assets. I had often heard that my character defects were good instincts gone awry, but it never quite registered. If they started out as assets, then why wouldn't God want to convert them back? Knowing that I could become the person I pretended to be filled me with peace. I no longer have to try to be "good." God does it for me.

My character defects surface on a daily basis. I love knowing that God transforms them—not to glorify me, but to do his bidding. Step Seven lays the foundation to work the rest of the Steps. When working with sponsees on Step Seven, I ask them to list their glaring character defects. Then together we list the assets into which God will transform them. It has become a beautiful piece of Step work for me. When just listing character defects seems too negative, looking at the positive— the asset side—gives us hope.

JUNE 24

"What all compulsive eaters have in common is that our bodies and minds seem to send us signals about food that are quite different from those the normal eater receives."

—*The Twelve Steps and Twelve Traditions of Overeaters Anonymous*, 2nd ed., p. 4

My diseased mind tries to tell me that by compulsively eating certain foods, I can make a situation better. I now know this is not true. I accept the fact that I react to food differently from normal eaters. I am different from a normal eater. I may also feel that my life is very different from my fellow OA members. Our compulsive eating may be the only thing we have in common, but that doesn't matter. Our desire to stop eating compulsively brings us together as one. Even the most different OA fellow shares my disease. Being part of the OA fellowship means that I never have to feel alone. My mind will never operate the way a normal eater's does. I accept the fact that I will always have this disease. However, now I no longer have to feel isolated, different, or ashamed. Today I can rest easy in the fact that I am not alone.

JUNE 25

"A person doesn't have to be abstinent to be welcome at OA meetings.… In fact, many of us have kept coming back to OA despite problems with abstinence and have found this to be the key to our recovery."

—*The Twelve Steps and Twelve Traditions of Overeaters Anonymous*, 2nd ed., pp. 108–109

I am thankful that OA doesn't base its membership requirements on weight, but only on a desire to stop eating compulsively. Sometimes I could only show up at a meeting and contribute to the Seventh Tradition. I cried, nodded, and tried to act as if everything was okay, even though I was falling apart emotionally.

By the grace of my God and my courage not to leave the rooms, something miraculous happened over time. I heard the message of those long-time abstaining members. It didn't happen that one day I did everything OA suggests, but slowly I started to ask the right people profound questions. This eventually led me to the one person who was willing and strong enough to overcome every obstacle I put up to resist recovery. It works, no matter what.

JUNE 26

"We learned we could 'act as if.'"

— *The Twelve Steps and Twelve Traditions of Overeaters Anonymous*, 2nd ed., p. 13

As a newcomer, I sometimes had difficulty accepting all that the program had to offer. Then I was told to "act as if" I did believe whatever I was having trouble accepting. There were times I couldn't even do that, and I would pray for the willingness to be able to "act as if." By learning this, I was able to open my mind to new ideas. Eventually I was able to stop acting, and really start believing. If we open our minds and hearts, we can begin the healing process that will bring us the peace and serenity we all deserve.

JUNE 27

"Welcome back. Welcome home!"
—*Welcome Back*, p. 11

These last four words of the *Welcome Back* pamphlet helped save my life.

Consumed by mental, emotional, physical, and spiritual pain, I returned to OA after a sixteen-year relapse. I thought only death would release me from this pain. Thoughts of suicide grew with the progressing, never-ceasing pain.

Even though I never told my husband about these thoughts, he worried about me and urged me to find help. I said I wanted to try Overeaters Anonymous again; if it had not developed into a "diet-and-calories club," I knew I would find help there. He said he didn't care where I went, that he only wanted his wife back. It was 1987, and the meeting I went to was a Big Book study meeting.

That meeting opened the door of hope. As I read the *Welcome Back* pamphlet, I touched the words "Welcome back, Welcome *home!*" and cried.

JUNE 28

"Surely it would be exaggerating to say we were incapable of managing our lives. We certainly could use some help with the compulsive eating, but with the rest of life, we were doing fine."

—*The Twelve Steps and Twelve Traditions of Overeaters Anonymous*, 2nd ed., p. 5

I bought into that idea at first. I had a respected career, managed a house, paid my bills, and basically thought I was Superwoman. How could this seemingly competent woman be incapable of managing her own life? When someone asked exactly what I had control over in my life, I was stumped. I certainly didn't control what went on at my job, what broke down at my house, or how others treated me. I suddenly found it difficult to find anything I really controlled. After this realization, I was able to turn my will and my life over to the care of my Higher Power. Now my life is much less stressful and chaotic. The little things don't worry me as much. Accepting that I am not in control is a very freeing experience. Today I admit I am not Superwoman, and I can't do it alone. I can trust that my Higher Power is taking care of me.

"Our purpose in doing Step Eight is not to judge others, but to learn attitudes of mercy and forgiveness."

—*The Twelve Steps and Twelve Traditions of Overeaters Anonymous*, 2nd ed., p. 59

An OA friend mailed me a sand dollar and an essay he had written on perfectionism. His writing helped me let go of this character defect. The essay says to look at the sand dollar. It's not broken, but it has flaws. It may be stained and have a nicked edge or a small hole. Can you still love it? If you can learn to love your imperfect sand dollar, you are capable of loving the imperfect world and people around you. People have disappointed you, hurt you, and let you down by being imperfect. Can you let go of the idea of perfection and accept reality, loving people just the way they are?

Love the imperfect people around you. Love your imperfect self and your imperfect world. For if you cannot love life the way it is, you will suffer from eternal loneliness. We all live in an imperfect world, surrounded by imperfect people. The ability to love yourself and those around you is a gift from God that enables you to live fully, bravely, and meaningfully in an imperfect world.

JUNE 30

"Hasn't this been our greatest problem: truly committing ourselves to refraining from compulsive eating on an ongoing basis? Full of determination, we are great in the short run, but when the boredom from the daily routine begins to set in, we lose interest....

A diet is something temporary.... Abstaining from compulsive eating, unlike dieting, has a sense of permanence about it. However, unlike our dieting days, we abstain only one day at a time."

—*A Lifetime of Abstinence: One Day at a Time*, p. 2

When first in OA, I didn't know what I should eat each day. I asked other OA members who were using a food plan what was working for them. One member simply replied, "I need to enjoy my food, because I'm eating today the way I will be eating for the rest of my life; it won't change someday." I found, too, through years of moderate eating one day at a time, that the weight did come off, without any hint of "dieting" behavior. In OA, I started to focus on the events of my life, which turned out to be much more interesting than watching my weight go up and down. In fact, because my weight was none of my business, it took care of itself.

JULY 1

"Humbly asked Him to remove our shortcomings."
—Step Seven

This, to me, was the true "action" Step. It required asking the Power outside of myself to change me, to make me something alien to myself. It required more trust than anything else I was asked to do and still demands trust as I continue to evolve into a new, unknown creation. This Step taught me humility, that state of being humble. Humble, according to the dictionary, is "the state of reflecting, expressing, or offering in a spirit of deference."

Before this Step, it was all about me—my powerlessness, my beliefs, my shortcomings, and my plans to resolve them. This Step changed all of that. The deference—"respect or esteem due to a superior"—clarified who was in power, who I should believe in, and the reason for giving over my shortcomings. It is all about becoming the person that my Higher Power needs me to be in order to carry out his will. That is what my program is about. With this Step I have surrendered my role as principal and joined the chorus of the Fellowship.

JULY 2

"From now on, we cease telling ourselves we are always going to be dishonest, selfish, abusive, stupid, or bad people. Instead, we repeatedly affirm the truth about ourselves—that we are becoming honest, caring, nurturing, wise, and effective human beings as we practice our new behaviors, day by day."

—*The Twelve Steps and Twelve Traditions of Overeaters Anonymous*, 2nd ed., p. 55

It is old behavior to berate myself for failing to perfectly work the Steps of the program. I learned that I cannot afford to continue doing this when I'm working Step Seven. Shaming myself for falling back into old behaviors is an old behavior in itself, and it helps keep me in all my character defects longer. The hours in my day become very precious upon entering OA. Haven't I suffered enough?

Working the first Six Steps to the best of my ability helps build a strong foundation to supply the humility I will need for Step Seven. I realize that I'm not the sickest or the healthiest person I know. I'm just about average. What a relief to also realize I will always be becoming a better person in OA. I will never arrive.

JULY 3

"Step Seven calls for us to adopt an attitude of humility."
—*The Twelve Steps and Twelve Traditions of Overeaters Anonymous*, 2nd ed., p. 51

I didn't think I could muster up the attitude of humility necessary to work Step Seven and to proceed. Then I realized that I first practiced humility by admitting powerlessness in Step One, by admitting insanity (Step Two), by letting God take control (Step Three), by admitting defects (Step Four), and then by sharing the defects (Step Five). So I have been practicing humility. I just hadn't tripped over the word "humbly" before. Since I have been granted humility all along, this evidence confirms that I will be granted enough to continue the path of the Twelve Steps.

JULY 4

"I finally understood that fighting the problem of compulsive overeating would never in this life relieve me of it."

—*For Today*, p. 96

I couldn't understand it! After maintaining a 100-pound weight loss for over two years, I relapsed and continued to relapse for the next seven years. After every regained abstinence, I'd share in meetings that I'd surrendered. Surrender, to me, meant "hitting bottom," praying desperately for help, then trying something different—food plan, sponsor, meetings—all external changes.

Today I know that this was not surrendering. I simply did what I needed to do to recover until I was no longer so desperate. A part of me always believed that someday I'd be able to eat normally. I still fought my food problem and other things in my life. Since I stopped fighting my Higher Power's will, one day at a time, I've not relapsed. My life has become more than "manageable." It has become more fulfilling than I could have ever imagined.

Someone once told me, "Life before surrender is a boxing match; after surrender it's surfing." Today, I'm gratefully and joyfully surfing.

JULY

"God grant me the serenity to accept the things I cannot change, courage to change the things I can, and wisdom to know the difference."

—Serenity Prayer

After more than a year in program, these words have become second nature to me; I have repeated them a thousand times. What an awakening for me one day as I said the prayer, hand in hand with my OA friends, and finally understood its simple message. Until then I had believed that I had to decide, with God's help, which of the people, places, and things in my life would benefit most from my interference. I now know that I am powerless over all of them. It is very simple. There is no decision to be made on my part. The things I cannot change are all the things outside of myself. The only thing I can change is myself. When I say the prayer, I am asking for the willingness to accept everything and the courage to change only myself. Only with the acceptance of this simple fact comes the serenity I seek.

JULY 6

"'You won't know that you have lived until you have lived this way.'"

—*Beyond Our Wildest Dreams*, p. 28

If someone had told me, six years before I came to OA, that I'd more than double my body weight, be riddled with fear and depression, and lose everything that mattered to me, I'd have said that was impossible. If someone had told me at my first meeting that in less than six years, I'd be eating healthy foods in healthy amounts at healthy times, have a normal body weight, be free of fear and depression, and be a brand-new person with a brand-new life, I'd have said that was impossible.

Many people settle for "okay." They just go through each day, often thinking in terms of problems, rather than solutions. We're the lucky ones. We've found time-tested solutions to any problem life could possibly bring. We've discovered what the Big Book calls "'a design for living'[2] that really works." It brings us a happy, joyous, and free abstinence and so much more. We don't have to settle for less than every single promise in the Big Book coming absolutely true!

---

[2] *Alcoholics Anonymous*, 4th ed., p. 28

JULY 7

"Humility is often considered the essence of Step Seven. Being humble might be defined as accepting things exactly as they are."

—*Sponsoring Through the Twelve Steps*, p. 14

How often did I blame other people for my overeating?

It seemed so real to say my parent forced me to eat compulsively. My history of inadequacy, fear, and shame appeared to be due to lack of "proper" love. My struggles with mental health problems could have been prevented if only "they" had been different.

Before I really worked the Seventh Step, I made the choice to dwell in self-centered thinking. Willingness to become humble and let God remove my defects has made all the difference. Serenity is a great exchange for giving up blaming.

JULY 8

"Clearly, if we are to live free of the bondage of compulsive eating, we must abstain from all foods and eating behaviors that cause us to eat compulsively."

— *The Twelve Steps and Twelve Traditions of Overeaters Anonymous*, 2nd ed., p. 4

When I was new to OA, my old ideas were usually 180 degrees from the things I heard at meetings and read in the literature. The idea of being in bondage to certain foods and eating behaviors was in striking contrast to my old idea that these foods and behaviors were "treats." The key for me was getting honest enough to acknowledge that they really were causing me problems.

At first, I tried to argue that I needed to eat this way because of my problems. But as I abstained one day at a time, I began to see those problems vanish from my life, sometimes quickly, sometimes slowly. And as this happened, I began to see the connection between my relationship to food and the problems. Now it begins to make sense: anything that causes problems in my life holds me in bondage. Abstinence opens that prison door and makes all of the miracles of recovery possible.

"We find it easier for each of us simply to be a part of the group. This is essential to recovery from our disease of isolation. It means supporting and being supported by our fellow OA members."

—*The Twelve Steps and Twelve Traditions of Overeaters Anonymous*, 2nd ed., p. 167

This passage tells me I have a disease of isolation, and the solution is to be part of the group. It also tells me that being part of the group means I support my fellow OA members, and they support me. When I first came to OA, I didn't feel "part of" anything in my life. I never felt that I belonged or fit in anywhere. OA tells me that I do belong because I am a compulsive overeater. It doesn't matter how much I weigh, how much money I earn, what color my hair is, or anything else. I belong and am equal in OA. I isolated because I was afraid to let anyone know me. Being a part of the group allowed me to open up a little at a time. As I felt more a part of the group, I felt more of the support available to me. From that, I learned to support others. Together we can do what we could never do alone.

JULY

"Some of us misunderstand this Step and act as if we can remove our shortcomings on our own."

—*The Twelve Steps and Twelve Traditions of Overeaters Anonymous*, 2nd ed., p. 47

I'm supposed to recognize that I am powerless over my character defects and turn them over to my Higher Power. I don't do this gracefully. Instead, I wrestle with my character defects. I drag them down into the mud. I struggle and groan and expend great amounts of energy fighting them. Only when I have no more energy left and I see that the character defect isn't even winded—in fact, doesn't even know it's been waging a war—do I admit I am powerless.

When my own best efforts to remove my character defects end in disaster, I can be open to the message that someone much more understanding and accepting of me than I am needs to take over handling my life. That's a tremendous relief.

JULY 11

"If we are to reach an informed decision, the group needs to take into account everybody's ideas. For this reason, OA groups give all viewpoints a full hearing—even minority viewpoints."

—*The Twelve Steps and Twelve Traditions of Overeaters Anonymous*, 2nd ed., p. 100

As a longtimer, I sometimes think I know what is best for OA. I've learned over the years to reserve a decision until all viewpoints are heard. Often the newcomer presents a view no one else has considered, and it changes everyone's mind. Our Traditions state that we make an informed group conscience. To be informed, we must listen to everyone. If we are always to keep the good of OA in mind, we must ensure that every viewpoint is heard with respect and compassion. We listen attentively and with an open mind. We can then make a decision based on what is best for our group and for OA as a whole.

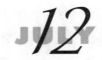
JULY 12

"And that truth—our promise of recovery—is in every OA meeting when we join hands, pray together, and joyously, lovingly encourage one another: Keep coming back!"

—*Overeaters Anonymous*, 3rd ed., p. 22

"Keep coming back!" We say it at the end of every meeting. But hearing those words in a new way helped bring me back from a long, painful relapse. I struggled so hard to regain my abstinence, to break my isolation, to redevelop a relationship with my Higher Power. But I seemed to always slip back into the grips of the disease. And then I heard, "Keep coming back" one day, and I made a decision to do just that. If I slipped away from my abstinence, I was determined to "keep coming back" to it. If I stopped talking to my Higher Power, I was determined to "keep coming back" to him. If I found I wasn't using the Tools or trying to work the Steps, I decided to "keep coming back" to them. It's not easy to "keep coming back" to the Principles of our program when the disease whispers in our ear that we're hopeless. But the decision to "keep coming back" has led me out of the despair and back into the light of recovery. Keep coming back—it works!

"Once we compulsive eaters truly take the Third Step, we cannot fail to recover."

—*The Twelve Steps and Twelve Traditions of Overeaters Anonymous*, 2nd ed., p. 23

Some mornings I awaken earlier than usual, my mind alive with frantic thoughts. The fear has returned. I will not get something that I want; things will not turn out well; my life has been reduced to keeping my disease at bay. These are the products of my self-centered fear: negativity, anxiety, living in a future not yet formed with an ungrateful heart. I see only what my disease has taken from me—everything that I "deserved."

I take my quiet time and begin to see new possibilities. I surrender the need to know how it will all turn out. I realize that I am getting well, a day at a time. I am learning how to trust. We who have been deeply affected by this disease band together to teach each other how to live without resorting to compulsive eating. I am exactly where I'm supposed to be. When I take my fear to God, he gives me the ability and the desire to see my life more clearly. My faith leads me to everything I need to surmount my difficulties if I am open to receiving the gift. I trust that God will take care of me.

JUL 14

> "By writing down our grievances, we place a boundary around them."
>
> —*The Twelve Steps and Twelve Traditions of Overeaters Anonymous*, 2nd ed., p. 61

Writing has been a part of my recovery from the beginning. I start my day with prayer on my knees, followed by writing. My writing is a continuation of my prayer time because it takes the form of a letter to my Higher Power. I lay out whatever is going on with me: my fears, my concerns, my questions, my failures, my successes.

Instead of thoughts floating around in my head with no beginning and no end, they assume shape and size when I write them down. More often than not, within a short time, I receive answers to my questions, comfort for my failures; in other words, whatever I need. My problems don't seem so large when they have boundaries. I gain new perspective on things and see solutions where before I only saw chaos. Today I am willing to spend fifteen minutes putting down on paper what is going on in my head so that I can see more clearly and gain sanity.

JULY 15

"*Many of us thought about suicide. Some of us tried it.*"

—*The Twelve Steps and Twelve Traditions of Overeaters Anonymous*, 2nd ed., p. 11

I used to change my mind (a lot!) about what and how much I would eat. Clearly, if I were to try suicide and wind up dead, there would be no changing my mind!

I would avoid making commitments because I could not count on myself to deliver. Or I would quickly make promises, force myself to keep them, but hate "being used."

I need to make plans and commitments, and I need to do it carefully. Then I need to do what I said that I would do. When I began committing my food to an OA sponsor and sticking to the commitment, a first benefit was greater confidence that I could make and keep other commitments, such as completing a task at work.

Today, I do plan my meals carefully, based both on what my body really needs and on what foods I will enjoy eating when mealtime comes. (No more "beating myself up" by planning disagreeable food to punish myself.) My self-esteem depends upon being able to make and keep commitments.

JULY 16

"Just for today I will have a quiet half hour all by myself and relax. During this half hour, sometime, I will try to get a better perspective on my life."

—Just For Today

Having recently become a stay-at-home mom, walking has become a great way for me to practice "quiet time." Getting out of my house helps me get out of my head and into a place where I am receptive to hearing my Higher Power speak to me.

First, I clear my head of all the clutter that has piled up from people, situations, and feelings. Sometimes I rant and rave, spilling my story out to God as I stomp my feet on the sidewalk. Sometimes, I apologize to God as I admit attitudes, thoughts, and actions that I'm experiencing or have already exposed other people to that were less than honorable. I then mentally list amends I need to make. At times, my heart sings out songs of praise as I breathe in the fresh air, listen to the birds, and realize the joy I feel inside just to be alive in this world today.

Then, I quiet my heart and am free to listen to what my God would say to me. Sometimes, he just soothes my feelings by allowing me to tenderly feel his love within the stillness of my heart. Sometimes he gives me the willingness and the courage to face people and situations with the truths I need to express to them. Always, I am refreshed and renewed for finishing my day without the need for overeating, secure in the knowledge that I am loved.

"Sought through prayer and meditation to improve our conscious contact with God ..."

—Step Eleven

After my first conscious contact with my Higher Power, I tried to reconnect and maintain that pink-cloud feeling. I couldn't do it for long. Usually I remembered to ask God for help after I had put my foot in my mouth, after I had done it my way, after I had tried everything else. I became humble when I could not do the thing I most wanted to do: to remember God in all my affairs. I believed in our program. What else is there for me? Humility, faith, and service kept me coming back for six years with no weight loss and sometimes with no consistent abstinence. The hope in the promises was there for me too. It had to be. Why do I have a clean, losing abstinence now? I stayed around until the miracle happened for me.

JULY 18

"Thank your Higher Power that you have found OA and no longer need to use food to solve your problems."

—*A Lifetime of Abstinence: One Day at a Time*, p. 4

I know many people who have spent years before dying attempting to find a label for their ailments. At least I know the name of the disease that has affected my life so drastically. Learning more about the various symptoms of food compulsion prepares me to take action to manage it through the Twelve Steps and OA's Tools of Recovery. The mental obsession, the cravings, the self-centeredness, the isolation, and the feelings of grandiosity make sense in the context of the disease.

Now when I feel angry, rejected, or depressed, I can look for perspective in the AA and OA literature. I identify with the thousands of recovering people who have suffered the same ills and who have found happiness and freedom from the bondage of compulsive eating.

What joy it is to have choices about my future, one day at a time.

JULY 19

> "If something has repeatedly worked well for us or for someone else in a similar situation, we may assume it will work in our present situation, ultimately bringing good to us and to others, which is God's will."

> —*The Twelve Steps and Twelve Traditions of Overeaters Anonymous*, 2nd ed., p. 22

I owe much of my recovery to the experiences voiced by others. I did not always believe that what worked for others would work for me. But loving OA members shared with me an approach they used with great success: their experience with "acting as if." By using this concept, I was able to develop trust in a Higher Power that was all-accepting, loving, and understanding. I "acted as if" until one day God actually was all these things to me. This approach also allowed me to achieve feelings of love and compassion toward my mother, where I once felt only emptiness.

I pray that I will always be teachable and open to the experience of others. Likewise, may God allow me to be a vehicle for his good works by sharing my own experience with another compulsive overeater.

"And the resentment that poisoned our hearts for years is washed away."

> —The Twelve Steps and Twelve Traditions of Overeaters Anonymous, 2nd ed., p. 63

At age forty-five, I had hated my father for most of my life. I didn't really remember why until recently, when a frivolous Sunday visit to a flea market (combined with an open mind about the amends segment of the OA program) revealed an unexpected opportunity to heal a lifelong and, in hindsight, unnecessary hurt.

That innocent afternoon, I disinterestedly chanced upon a coin vendor marketing his wares. I hadn't collected coins since the childhood occasion when my father had spent my collection at face value. Then I saw it, the war nickel that I had always dreamed would be worth millions one day and that my father had stolen from me. This coin was in approximately the same condition as the one I had lost. I nervously asked the price and bought it for a quarter!

I realized then that I had hated my own father, all my life—for twenty-five cents. I started to cry, then laugh, then cry, then laugh, then cry…! Somehow the tears and laughter washed away the hate and anger planted so long ago and nurtured so carefully by my disease. I call it my two-bit resentment!

Today, with the help of OA and the Twelve Steps, I live in reality and truly avoid making situations larger than they really are.

JULY 21

"Often we caused ourselves problems because we didn't realize that there were some foods and eating behaviors we could handle comfortably and some we couldn't."

—*The Twelve Steps and Twelve Traditions of Overeaters Anonymous*, 2nd ed., p. 19

This saying creates an image of the balance between my Higher Power's part and my part in any life situation. And "balance" is the elusive "sanity" referred to in Step Two: "Came to believe that a Power greater than ourselves could restore us to sanity." So often in my disease I have used "magical thinking," hoping that a situation would resolve itself. Yet other times I have "over-rowed," without benefit or direction from God as a compass.

When it came to physical recovery and adopting a plan of eating, I had always tried what someone else was doing. Experience eventually taught me that other people's food plans did not work for me. The compulsion stayed with me until I prayed to be led to the plan of eating that would work best for me. Then I prayed for the willingness to row the boat, to take action with a plan of eating one meal, one day at a time. As a result, I have been attending OA, free of the compulsion, for almost a year.

JULY 22

"Abstinence can help reverse the devastating effects of this disease and restore balance to mind, body, and spirit."

—*A Lifetime of Abstinence: One Day at a Time*, p. 8

I seem to have such a limited ability to relate my actions to their consequences. Coming into OA I blamed my weight on everything but my eating—my family, society, my metabolism. By the grace of my Higher Power, I finally saw the relationship between my eating behaviors and my weight. Abstinence brought weight loss. But over time, I experienced slips and eventually a relapse.

Lately I've realized that when I'm abstinent, I feel good; when I'm into the food, my life is unmanageable. This connection has been there all the time, but the only part of it I had made was that abstinence brought weight loss. I am finally understanding that for me, staying abstinent means the simple ability to eat and sleep normally and wake up glad I am alive, glad I abstained yesterday, and glad I have the privilege of abstaining today. Each morning I make a point of remembering that the reason I feel good, the reason I sleep well, and the reason I'm glad I am alive is because I am abstinent. I was abstinent yesterday, and I have a choice to accept the privilege of abstaining today. Finally, this connection is clicking into place. I am so grateful.

I see that abstinence is the foundation underlying my ability to appreciate all that is good in my life. Today I choose to abstain from compulsive eating.

"For many of us, this freedom came when we took Step Three and turned the entire problem over to our Higher Power."

— *The Twelve Steps and Twelve Traditions of Overeaters Anonymous*, 2nd ed., p. 18

The Twelfth Step of Overeaters Anonymous talks about the qualities we gain as a result of working the Twelve Steps, but the word freedom appears so many times in all of our literature, I began to think about the freedoms from my disease I gained by working each of the Steps of Overeaters Anonymous:

One: Freedom from the obsession with food

Two: Freedom from insanity and hopelessness

Three: Freedom from the bondage of self

Four: Freedom from dishonesty

Five: Freedom from isolation

Six: Freedom from running the show

Seven: Freedom from self-reliance

Eight: Freedom from blame

Nine: Freedom from fear of people

Ten: Freedom from complacency

Eleven: Freedom from loneliness

Twelve: Freedom from lack of purpose

"It is important to bear in mind that knowledge of ourselves and our nutritional needs is useless without the kind of help we find through working all of OA's Twelve Steps."

—*The Twelve Steps and Twelve Traditions of Overeaters Anonymous*, 2nd ed., p. 20

I have to remind myself of this every day. It is easy to see OA as another way of losing weight, a means of learning some more tricks. When sponsoring people, I also need to find a balance: a focus on what they have learned that day about themselves, food, and nutrition, and a focus on how a Power greater than themselves is helping them get well. It's about reminding myself that this is a three-fold program—physical, emotional, and spiritual.

"We have what we need any time we are willing to let go of self-will and humbly ask for help."

—*The Twelve Steps and Twelve Traditions of Overeaters Anonymous*, 2nd ed., p. 23

This seems to be the key to the program and to life: being able to let go of self-will and to reach out to a Power greater than myself for help. It took me many years in the program to feel that this is how it works. Self-will always seemed such a source of energy. Yet I couldn't see that this type of energy resulted in a lot of restlessness. There is much more peace in doing the things my Higher Power wants me to do. And, to my surprise, this doesn't mean things don't get done. I still do the laundry, have a job, cook a healthy meal. It's just my frame of mind that has changed.

JULY 26

"Our commitment to abstinence from compulsive eating is vital to our lives."

—*A Lifetime of Abstinence: One Day at a Time*, p. 6

Every morning I remind myself of my priorities. Abstinence is more important than anything else. I apply it in all areas. Abstinence is a higher priority than my family. Without it, I'm no good to my family anyway. Abstinence is a higher priority than my work. If I'm not abstinent, then my work isn't going to go as well. I can make all the money I want, but if I don't have abstinence, I'm never going to enjoy it. Abstinence helps me stay in the present. I am better able to develop that relationship with my Higher Power, and that's what OA is all about.

"We admitted we were powerless over food—that our lives had become unmanageable."

—Step One

As I was preparing my food one day, struggling to "get it right," "figure it out," and "control it," I recognized that "control is not one of the promises." I am, and always will be, powerless over my food, my thinking, and my life. All my attempts at control have brought me to the same place over and over again—loss of control. That's what all my days of dieting had been about. I was OA's equivalent to a dry drunk.

There is a Power, whom I choose to call God, that can restore me to sanity, sobriety, and abstinence. I cannot do that myself, any more than I can remove my character defects. Working the Twelve Steps is about learning to accept the gifts of willingness, surrender, sanity, serenity, and humility from my Higher Power. God is doing for me what I cannot do for myself so that I can carry that message to those still suffering. I can't keep my program unless I give it away; I can't give it away unless I accept it.

JULY 28

"Genuine humility brings an end to the feelings of inadequacy, the self-absorption, and the status seeking. Humility, as we encounter it in our OA Fellowship ... places us exactly where we belong, on an equal footing with our fellow beings and in harmony with God."

—*The Twelve Steps and Twelve Traditions of Overeaters Anonymous*, 2nd ed., p. 52

In my compulsive eating days, I rarely experienced humility. I compared myself to others and felt that I didn't measure up, that I wasn't good enough. I even confused this low opinion of myself with humility. These feelings led me straight to the food.

Working this program, I am learning to accept myself for who I am. I strive daily to let go of comparisons and have become more accepting of myself and others. I find comfort in the belief that my Higher Power's will for me each day includes being the best person that I can be. Best of all, the more truly and deeply I believe that I am okay, the more happy and serene I feel.

JULY 29

"I have found freedom."
　　　　—*For Today*, p. 252

On my bike ride I see the tower of the state prison far in the distance. I am reminded of the freedom I have from the prison of compulsive overeating. I am grateful that I have recovery but am mindful that the disease is always there, on the horizon. OA is a spiritual program. It means living a spiritual life. Recovery comes and remains by being faithful to surrender, prayer, and meditation on a daily basis. Each day I need to renew my commitment to abstinence, live the Twelve Steps, and follow my food plan. Only by doing this can I be confident that compulsive overeating will remain in the far distance.

JULY 30

"... a loving witness, someone who can keep our confidences and listen without judging us or seeking to fix us."

—*The Twelve Steps and Twelve Traditions of Overeaters Anonymous*, 2nd ed., p. 42

Someone who doesn't judge—I was not accustomed to that before OA. What a wonderful difference it is to find people who really listen to me! What a talent they have for listening and not attempting to solve my problems.

Can I also learn to do this? Why not? If I can work the Steps in the footsteps of my sponsor and others in the program, I can also learn to listen. Slowly, this ability is coming to me. I no longer plan what I am going to say while you are speaking. I actually strive to hear the feelings behind your words. The words themselves are not as important as the feelings conveyed.

Discovering people who listen to me is one of the many gifts of the program. And it is one that I can pass on to others. God has blessed me with many gifts since I walked through the doors of OA. The ability to be a loving witness is but one of them.

JULY 31

"Relapse is not inevitable."
   —*A New Plan of Eating*, p. 11

I had such a history of relapse that my sponsor said, "If nothing changes, nothing changes." That meant drastic change in every area of my life—one day at a time. My life was permeated by bad habits. Breaking bad habits can require lots of prayer and willingness. At first, just driving past the restaurant or grocery store and heading for a safe place took every ounce of willingness I could muster. But every time I do that, it gets easier the next time.

Just for today, I can do this. All of the power of the universe is behind every prayer, every attempt to do things a little bit better today than I did yesterday. It really is a new day. I now know what works and what doesn't. I can, for today, be kind to myself and to my body. I can be my own best friend. Even if I am taking baby steps in the direction of my dreams, I will get there.

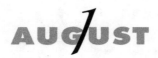

AUGUST 1

"As long as we have not forgiven people for harms they have done to us, we will find it impossible to make sincere amends to them for our side of the conflicts."

—The Twelve Steps and Twelve Traditions of Overeaters Anonymous, 2nd ed., p. 60

For me the essential element in Step Eight is forgiveness. Until I learned how to forgive, I could not even see where I was at fault.

I was not aware of the deep resentment I had against my parents for the abuse I endured as a child. My insecurities, fear of rejection, and low self-worth were all a direct result of suppressing those feelings. I began to truly search my past, and the old memories of abuse returned. As I examined them, hate, humiliation, and deep rage boiled out of me in floods of tears. I knew I could not forgive these wrongs myself, especially where my own defiance was often at fault.

It suddenly occurred to me to pray for a "spirit" of forgiveness. Gradually a peace enfolded me. Forgiveness came, and with it came complete deliverance from those damaged feelings. From that moment, I was healed. Once the miracle of forgiveness occurred, the amends happened naturally.

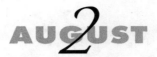
AUGUST 2

"As we become aware of what our healthy eating guidelines should be, we ask God for the willingness and the ability to live within them each day. We ask and we receive, first the willingness, and then the ability. We can count on this without fail."

—The Twelve Steps and Twelve Traditions of Overeaters Anonymous, 2nd ed., p. 21

One night at a Step-study meeting, I read the above passage and realized I had no ability to stay sober. Even if I prayed for willingness, my ability to live within my eating guidelines was zero. However, these words gave me a set of actions to take daily, trusting my Higher Power to do the rest. So I got on my knees and asked for the willingness and the ability to live within my eating guidelines and to practice the Twelve Steps for that day. Since then I've discovered that I can count on it without fail—one day, one minute at a time.

AUGUST 3

"'After all, nobody expects us to be perfect,' we say. 'We strive for progress, not perfection.' Such reasoning only delays our recovery. The Sixth Step calls for us to be entirely ready to have God remove all our defects of character. Those of us who take this Step with the total commitment required to make it work do indeed strive for the ultimate refinement of our character."

—The Twelve Steps and Twelve Traditions of Overeaters Anonymous, 2nd ed., p. 47

In Step Six, I use love, insight, and vision to release my current identity and self-image and open myself to further growth and recovery. I remember my ideals and dreams, and I pay attention to them. The Sixth Step is not about being controlled or coerced toward perfection, as my disease would have me believe. Rather, I prepare to become lighter: more fully me, more fully aware and living in my heart's desire. I envision a new self, with the intention of letting my Higher Power and my experiences bring me closer to who I really am. While this is, at times, a gradual and contemplative process, I am also in the Sixth Step any time I approach my life with openness to what the moment may show me.

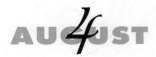
AUGUST 4

"Were entirely ready to have God remove all these defects of character."

—Step Six

Step Six is about change. It reminds me of a broken arm that had been set improperly, still defective and practically useless. A good surgeon could carefully re-break that arm and reset it so it would function perfectly. However, such an operation would be quite painful and could require many months to heal.

Step Six suggests removing old, destructive habits. One of my old habits was eating food that would "stick to my ribs." I also experienced dramatic emotional swings.

It has taken many years to change old eating habits and emotional reactions. But my Higher Power was the very skilled surgeon, and he was helped by the members of Overeaters Anonymous. Though the process was often painful, it resulted in a useful, happy life. I have learned that when the pain of where I am is worse than the fear of where I'm going, I welcome change.

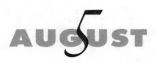

AUGUST 5

"Humility, as we encounter it in our OA Fellowship, places us neither above nor below other people on some imagined ladder of worth. It places us exactly where we belong, on an equal footing with our fellow beings."

—*The Twelve Steps and Twelve Traditions of Overeaters Anonymous*, 2nd ed., p. 52

Before I came to OA, my self-esteem swung wildly—from exceedingly low to arrogantly high. Usually I thought of myself as ugly, deeply flawed, and unlovable. Sometimes I tried to put myself above people I knew; I worked hard to convince myself and others that I was smarter or nicer, kinder, or more competent.

OA has helped me understand that humility means recognizing the equality of all persons. We are unique individuals with unique strengths and weaknesses. We each have gifts to offer. We are all valuable human beings, worthy of respect. In my journey of recovery, I am called to be the best person I can be and to respect others for who they are. As I work toward those goals, I become truly equal and in harmony with life.

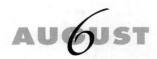

AUGUST 6

"Compulsive eating and compulsive food behaviors are removed on a daily basis ... achieved through the process of surrendering."

—*Overeaters Anonymous*, 3rd ed., p. 3

Surrendering my worries and concerns about other people and everyday living was relatively easy for me and brought me serenity and peace. However, I found it much harder to surrender food and its over-consumption to my Higher Power. I was unwilling to give up the comfort and relaxation that food gave me. I did not trust that I would find comfort and relaxation without food. The few days of abstinence that I was able to put together finally showed me that I was relaxed and comfortable on those days.

This discovery led me to the realization that my Higher Power gives me the gift of comfort and peace one day at a time. Each day I have to surrender my food and my disease to God, and each day I'm able to relax without food. Each day I find comfort in all God's creations that I dismissed when I took comfort only from food.

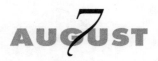

AUGUST 7

> *"We shouldn't be surprised or discouraged if we have an occasional, sudden desire to eat outside of our food plan. As disturbing as these cravings and thoughts may be, it is important to remember that we* do not need to act on them!*"*
>
> —*A Lifetime of Abstinence: One Day at a Time*, p. 6

When I first came to OA, it was incredibly comforting to read those words. You mean it was actually normal for me to suddenly crave food for no apparent reason? Someone pointed out that if it was always easy, very few OA members would keep coming back. All right, but what about those terrifying food nightmares I'd have, when I'd wake up convinced I'd binged? A very helpful sponsor turned those dreams from negatives to plusses for me by calling them "freebies"—opportunities to experience all the horrible feelings accompanying a binge— regret, self-hatred, terror—without having to actually go through it. What a relief I get from the literature and wise words of other OA members' soothing reminders that whatever I'm feeling is perfectly okay.

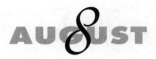

AUGUST 8

"… restore us to sanity."

—Step Two

When I first came into program eighteen years ago, I skipped over some Steps. These were Steps I thought I had already completed. Step Two was one of these. For instance, I already believed, so there was nothing more to think through—and so, onto Step Three.

A couple of years later (and add one awful relationship mess), I was going through the Steps again, and this time it was not simply a head exercise, but rather one involving my entire life, inside and out.

One day, during this crisis time, I walked into a local art gallery, something I was not normally inclined to do. I stopped to watch in awe as a woman behind the counter was restoring a painting. I was completely taken by her care-filled movements as she worked.

This image stayed with me, and the next day as I was doing my early morning lotion and moisturizer routines, it occurred to me that I was my Higher Power's artistic creation. My Higher Power was now restoring me through my Step work with the same care and knowledge that the artist used to restore her painting in the gallery. My entire Step Two task was to believe that I, too, could be restored through my care tasks—be they writing, going to meetings, taking quiet time, or phone time with my sponsor—and be a participant in this great restoration work. There was nothing to skip over any longer in Step Two.

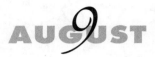

AUGUST 9

"Those of us who live this program don't simply carry the message; we are the message."

—*The Twelve Steps and Twelve Traditions of Overeaters Anonymous*, 2nd ed., pp. 86–87

I don't just work the program; I live it. That means I try to incorporate all Twelve Steps into my daily life. After practicing for many years, the practice has become a habit. The more habitual it becomes, the easier it is to live the program. It becomes second nature; I don't have to think about it. That means I am a message of recovery for those who still suffer. I live this program for me, for my peace of mind, and for my sanity. That I am a message for others is a gift from God. I am an example that "keep coming back" works!

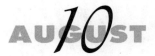

AUGUST 10

"We now say yes to this Power, deciding from here on to follow spiritual guidance in making every decision."

— The Twelve Steps and Twelve Traditions of Overeaters Anonymous, 2nd ed., p. 18

In every decision? My mind went into instant rebuff mode upon reading those words. Oh sure, I could see the need to surrender my will and my life to a Power greater than myself in food-related matters. Just how many fruits can I dice up really small and cram on top of my cereal and still remain spiritually fit? How many trips to the salad bar constitutes a normal meal?

But every decision? Whether to ask for a raise, to take on a new sponsee, to read *Lifeline* or *TV Guide*, to go to bed with this attractive stranger, to phone my mother or my sponsor, to tell this jerk I'm plenty miffed—in all the small and large decisions that make up a day, that make up a life.

The words on the first page of Step Three gazed back at me serenely. I hesitated and then totally capitulated to their injunction. And I've never regretted that surrender.

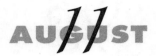

AUGUST 11

"I study the Big Book and OA materials, and I live in an 'attitude of gratitude' for the miracle of Overeaters Anonymous."

—*Abstinence*, 2nd ed., p. 10

An attitude of gratitude serves me best. Sometimes, though, I forget that gratitude is a choice. I can get caught up in negativity, resentments, or complaining. At these times, I am focusing on the way things should be according to me! These attitudes eat away at my abstinence. I am thankful today that I can recognize the danger of an attitude of resentment. Today I know there is nothing about which to be negative, resentful, or complaining that makes it worth breaking my abstinence. Nothing! Every blessing, however, is noteworthy because it will strengthen my abstinence. I am thankful today that I can choose gratitude. In doing so, my blessing list grows, and I can actually enjoy life instead of grumbling my way through it. Thank you, God, for abstinence, for gratitude.

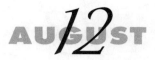

"Just staying abstinent—if it's all I can do today—is reaching for recovery."

—*For Today*, p. 167

Abstinence is where my recovery begins. That is the "food" I need to reach for. That is where insanity ends and serenity begins. Once I got a "taste" of serenity, I wanted more and more. The feeling of freedom from food is incredible. I have learned to ask for help from God, my sponsor, and my group. I have learned to tackle new problem foods in order to get more recovery. What I want to reach for now is not more food, but more recovery. Am I calling someone? Am I getting to meetings? Am I praying daily? Am I being grateful in prayer? Am I reading? Am I working the Steps? Am I asking God to make me willing? When tempted, I ask God to help me reach for more recovery instead of more food.

AUGUST 13

"By following these Steps, thousands of OA members have stopped eating compulsively. ...

What we do have to offer is far greater ... a Fellowship in which we find and share the healing power of love."

— The Twelve Steps and Twelve Traditions of Overeaters Anonymous, 2nd ed., p. 1

It is sometimes asked which is more important, the Steps or the Fellowship? For me the answer is that the Steps and the Fellowship are like two oars in a rowboat. If I only row with one arm I will go around in circles.

Before I was an OA member, I had a copy of the Twelve Steps on my wall. With great enthusiasm I went around making amends and went home to overeat. I'm glad to say I found healing power in the OA Fellowship. On the other hand, I have a friend who loved to socialize after meetings but thought the Steps were optional. She couldn't stay abstinent until she embraced the Steps. Today, we are both among the thousands of OA members who have many years of freedom from compulsive eating.

With one hand rowing the Steps and the other hand rowing the Fellowship, I have no free hands with which to overeat. God is on board, directing me to the dry land of a contented abstinence.

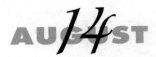
AUGUST 14

"Here, we experience the great truth that when we let go of our need to control people and simply allow our Higher Power to serve others through us we receive an abundance of joy and strength."

—The Twelve Steps and Twelve Traditions of Overeaters Anonymous, 2nd ed., p. 86

Allowing God to serve others through me has become the central purpose of my life. Practicing these Principles in all my affairs has not always been easy. I practiced first in OA meetings, then with OA friends, and then at work. The hardest place to practice these Principles has been at home, with my family. When I remember that my purpose is to allow God to serve others through me, my relationships are easier, my work life is a pleasure, and my home life is a joy. I no longer have to control people or situations. I trust God and focus on service.

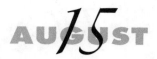

AUGUST 15

"Meetings are gatherings of two or more compulsive overeaters who come together to share their personal experience and the strength and hope OA has given them."

—*The Tools of Recovery*, p. 2

Life on life's terms can make my day feel chaotic, so it is a relief to walk into a meeting and hear the same comforting, familiar slogans from friends each week.

However, I've come to love OA meetings for their unpredictability, as well as their structure. Meetings are like jazz improvisation—never the same twice. Meetings have the unpredictability, freshness, and originality that almost make them an art form. When I come to OA meetings, I never know who will show up, what will be said, if newcomers will be there, or even if the group conscience will be followed.

Meetings happen exactly as they are supposed to; there are no accidents. They have a life of their own, run by a Power greater than ourselves. I can let go of the need to control meetings. My only responsibility is to show up and share honestly about my recovery.

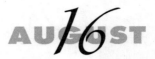

"The problem is with the control of food. Is one preoccupied with controlling food intake to the point that it's interfering with one's life? Just as being an alcoholic is not related to the amount one drinks, being a compulsive overeater is not related to the amount one weighs."

—*Overeaters Anonymous*, 3rd ed., p. 196

The disease makes me preoccupied with food, body image, weight, and control issues. I spent years thinking that if I just looked a certain way, ate certain things, and avoided eating certain things, I could be happy despite any problems life threw my way. I thought the reason I didn't have a life was because I was fat. Obsessing about these things, however, kept me from having a life. The fat was only the physical manifestation of the cocoon I had built to isolate myself from the pain of living.

What I really needed was a Higher Power to control my life and help me deal with my feelings, fears, and insecurities. It wasn't until I gave up trying to control what I ate that I noticed that I have a life to live, and it is a good one. Today I give my life to God, trusting him to lead me toward what he wants me to do, be, and experience. I thank God for loving me and pray that he will help me love myself.

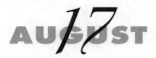

AUGUST 17

"In OA, we share a belief that we can each recover through a spiritual relationship with a Power that is greater than ourselves alone."

> —The Twelve Steps and Twelve Traditions of Overeaters Anonymous, 2nd ed., p. 75

The variety of religious, non-religious, and irreligious backgrounds in OA is truly impressive. We don't have to agree to disagree. What we all agree on is a reliance on a power that can relieve us, one day at a time, of this horrible disease. Relief from the burdens of compulsive overeating is only the beginning. Step Eleven is both a practical necessity and a spiritual dream come true.

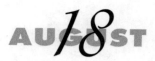

AUGUST 18

"Some of us have looked for help from qualified professionals."
—*The Twelve Steps and Twelve Traditions of Overeaters Anonymous*, 2nd ed., p. 43

Becoming abstinent and working the Steps brought my deeper psychological problems to the surface, so my sponsor suggested that I seek outside help. I was blessed to find a therapist who was also a member of a Twelve Step program. I learned that by using the Principles of the program in tandem with therapy, the favorable results multiplied.

Before each session I would pray, "God, I am powerless over my emotional and mental state. Please guide and direct this session. Give me the courage to speak my truth without censoring. Provide my therapist with the knowledge and insight that will best facilitate my recovery. Allow me to hear and accept these truths; guide me to the actions I need to take and provide me the willingness to take them. Thank you."

In time I was able to reach into the darkest corners of my soul and reveal the truth of my life: I came to OA as a victim; through OA and therapy discovered I was a survivor; today I am a thriver who enjoys a life of sane and happy usefulness.

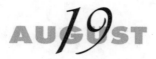
AUGUST 19

"Each day that we live well, we are well."

—*The Twelve Steps and Twelve Traditions of Overeaters
Anonymous*, 2nd ed., p. 87

What a change in attitude it has taken for me to recognize a
well-lived day and be grateful for it. Today, a day is well-lived
if I am abstinent by the grace of my Higher Power and this
Fellowship and if I have acted courteously and kindly toward
myself and others, so I owe no amends.

I am not perfect and have had slip-ups with food behaviors,
but I know the OA program has what I need to live well. By
continuing to work the Steps systematically, I am learning
more and more to accept and love myself just as I am—
imperfect, but progressing. I can forgive myself for making
mistakes and ask for my Higher Power's help to move on
and do the daily footwork of this program, letting go of
expectations and outcomes. I know I have lived well in a day
when I can see a long list of things to be grateful for, including
abstinence.

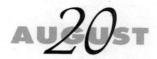

AUGUST 20

"*Abstinence is a country whose beauty and variety I could not have imagined in my most indulgent dreams.*"

—*For Today*, p. 71

When I am abstinent, I feel emotions that are sometimes uncomfortable, but bearable without excess food. I also keep my commitments most of the time; an interesting fact is I find I don't make very many commitments I don't want to keep. But whether my emotions are up or down, and whether my commitments are pleasant or not, I'm present for them.

When eating compulsively, I'm not present for or in the life I'm passively moving through. When abstinent, I'm present for and in a life I'm actively living. The landscape is varied. The terrain is challenging. The colors are glorious. Thank you, Higher Power, for a gift much greater than abstinence—the gift of life.

"The basic concept of Overeaters Anonymous is that compulsive overeating is a disease that affects the person on three levels— physical, spiritual, and emotional."

—*Overeaters Anonymous*, 3rd ed., p. 198

Recognition that compulsive overeating is a disease eased my guilty feelings that my inability to control my weight was a moral failure. My understanding of the three affected areas, and the importance of balance in recovery, was aided by a shared example of a three-legged stool. Having watched my uncle milk cows using such a stool, I could see how precarious the sitting would be if one leg were missing or shorter or longer than the others. This helped me see the importance of balance in these areas of my life as well. When my food is troubling me, I know that emotional and spiritual problems are also involved. Getting my feelings in the open by writing or sharing with trusted others, as well as prayer and meditation, have helped the considerable amount of recovery I have been given—physically, emotionally, and spiritually. Thank you, OA!

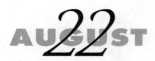

AUGUST 22

"If you hate a person, you hate something in him that is part of yourself. What isn't part of ourselves doesn't disturb us."

—Hermann Hesse as quoted in *For Today*, p. 158

"I hate when you speak to me like that." "I hate when you don't call me back right away." These are phrases I previously used. I did not accept others; I thought I knew how others should act.

When I started going to meetings, reading literature, and talking to others in OA, I found out it was me who had the problems. I had shortcomings that I was not willing to accept, so I criticized those around me.

Slowly, in finding compassion myself, I have grown to accept others. I have learned through OA to see each individual as a unique and wonderful human being—I have even learned that about me! I know when I criticize someone else's habits I must look within and see what part of me I am not accepting fully. I take time out for a mental inventory, journal writing, or talking with my sponsor.

This new way of living has saved my life, and for that I am grateful every single day!

AUGUST 23

"Once we compulsive eaters truly take the Third Step, we cannot fail to recover."

—*The Twelve Steps and Twelve Traditions of Overeaters Anonymous*, 2nd ed., p. 23

This sentence kept alive in me the hope that I could recover from compulsive overeating. It kept me coming back, even through the tough times. It kept me coming back when I felt unloved. It kept me coming back because I knew something had not yet "clicked" for me. But I believed that as long as I kept trying and working the program to the best of my ability, I would be "clicked" into a new dimension.

Abstinence has not come easily for me. Many times it eluded me, and even after several years in OA, I have times of relapse. Many times I felt that sustained abstinence from compulsive overeating was impossible for me, despite the fact that I believed I had made great headway on the spiritual and emotional levels. I have received many gifts as a result of working this program; one of the greatest gifts was hope. Without hope, I could easily have given up and eaten myself into mindless oblivion.

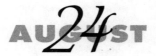

"We ask and we receive, first the willingness, and then the ability. We can count on this without fail."

> —*The Twelve Steps and Twelve Traditions of Overeaters Anonymous*, 2nd ed., p. 21

The first time someone in OA suggested that I needed to pray for willingness, I thought they were crazy. I was overweight, had tried many diets, and hated myself. How could I not be willing to be thin? Then I began observing my behavior. I prayed for God to keep me from eating my binge foods. I ate food that had fallen into the trash. I ate food that I knew was addictive. Then came the realization: I was not willing.

Okay, God, now I am willing to pray for the willingness. Praying for willingness has made a difference. The ability came slowly as I became willing to find a healthy way of eating. It came as I became willing to reach out and ask for help with my isolation. It came as I became willing to humble myself and surrender my powerlessness over food. It came as I worked the program one day at a time.

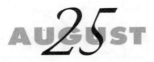
AUGUST 25

"No longer will we allow fear to keep us from doing what is best for us."

—*The Twelve Steps and Twelve Traditions of Overeaters Anonymous*, 2nd ed., pp. 48–49

I relapsed after more than two years of solid abstinence. My compulsion found many reasons for this other than the real ones: fear and lack of trust in my Higher Power. Fear kept me from moving ahead in my program. Fear made me feel disconnected and resentful. Fear made me heavier than I had ever been before. Fear made me hopeless. But I kept going to meetings.

My new sponsor had twelve years of abstinence. She had what I wanted. She encouraged me to attend ninety meetings in ninety days, and I began hearing the message daily. Finally, after some willingness, self-trust, and honesty, I began to understand my relapse. The belief that my Higher Power would not take care of me during Steps Six and Seven threw me into relapse. I had decided, unconsciously, that the pain of compulsive overeating was less than the pain of growth.

Today I am abstinent. I choose the pain of growth because I trust that my Higher Power will care for me no matter what the outcome.

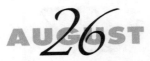

AUGUST 26

"In OA, we share a belief that we can each recover through a spiritual relationship with a Power that is greater than ourselves alone."

—*The Twelve Steps and Twelve Traditions of Overeaters Anonymous*, 2nd ed., p. 75

When I read this sentence, a sense of security settles over me. Here in one sentence is the essence of our wonderful program. I can reflect on all the methods I previously tried to control my compulsive eating. In spite of great emotional resolve and physical need, nothing worked over the long haul. Yes, I lost weight. No, I did not change my thinking.

It was not until I brought a Higher Power (whom I choose to call my God) into my equation that I began to experience physical, emotional, and spiritual recovery. Although I cannot pinpoint the time when I converted from dieting to working a spiritually-based program, it occurred as a result of working the Steps and using the Tools of the program daily. My reward for these efforts is fifteen years of abstinence, health, and happiness.

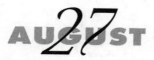
AUGUST 27

"We were left without faith that God could restore us to sanity about food."

> —*The Twelve Steps and Twelve Traditions of Overeaters Anonymous*, 2nd ed., p. 14

Over the years, I've relapsed periodically, never thinking of it as a rejection of my Higher Power. But it was. I was telling my Higher Power that I had more faith in food than in him. It was easier to drown my fears in food than to trust my Higher Power to carry me through them. It was easier to believe that God was too busy to care what I ate than to believe that he grieved over every extra bite I took.

One day I realized my lack of faith when I looked down at my plate, feeling an overwhelming sense of fear and panic. There was not enough food! My doubt in my Higher Power became obvious to me. How could I believe he would let me suffer hunger—hunger of the spirit, the mind, and the body? Since then I put my food and faith in God's hands and my old enemy, the disease, weakens on a daily basis.

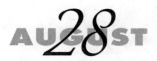

AUGUST 28

"What all compulsive eaters have in common is that our bodies and minds seem to send us signals about food that are quite different from those the normal eater receives."

—The Twelve Steps and Twelve Traditions of Overeaters Anonymous, 2nd ed., p. 4

Acceptance of being different from other people can be difficult, but it is also a relief. Before OA, I assumed that everyone experienced the same thoughts and feelings about food that I did, and that normal eaters were better people than I because they could resist excess food. This passage teaches me that they don't receive the same signals about food in the first place, so there is nothing for them to resist!

It is also a relief to learn that the sense of deprivation I sometimes experience when refraining from excess food is only an illusion. The faulty signals I receive about food—that it will make me feel better or fulfill my needs—are just that, faulty signals. There is no real deprivation in abstaining from excess foods or foods that will harm me. True deprivation is how I lived before OA—in bondage to food and fat.

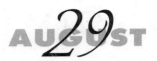

AUGUST 29

"We will love you until you can love yourself."

—program slogan

When I first came to Overeaters Anonymous, I could not fathom feeling truly loved by another. I felt unlovable. On the surface I acted as if I believed that others loved me, but inside I truly believed that if anyone really got to know me, they would find me unacceptable. Each time I called my sponsor, and she acted genuinely glad to hear from me, I cried. I wondered how she could care for someone like me. I thought there must be something wrong with her. When I went to meetings, people clapped when I shared. They dropped what they were doing to talk to me when I called them on the phone.

Listening to them share their difficulties made me realize that I was not so different and unacceptable. After all, I loved them. Could it be that I was lovable too? Slowly over time, with the help of my OA family and my relationship with my Higher Power, I began to feel lovable. Soon I began to treat myself like others were treating me. The miracle was happening. Through being loved, I am now able to love myself.

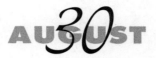

AUGUST 30

"If I don't know which way to go, I turn the problem over to God in steps three and eleven, completely confident that the answer will come."

—*For Today*, p. 25

Soon after I found OA, a woman at my home meeting stood up and said, "Last night the phone rang, and by the time I hung up, I was crazy. So I said a prayer, turned it over, and was free to enjoy the next three hours until dinner time."

The next day, driving to work, I noticed my mind racing over and over on the same problem. I said, "God, take this problem from me, and don't give it back unless I need to do something about it." It was hard to trust God to give it back if and when I needed to act on it, so I said, "I trust you, God."

God took it, and I was free to enjoy my ride. I have done that many times since then, and I don't think God has given very many of those problems back to me. They must have solved themselves. What freedom!

AUGUST 31

"My best thinking got me into trouble. I could 'think' my life to suit me; the only problem was that it didn't work."

—*For Today*, p. 298

In order to recover, I had to let go of my thinking and embrace believing. This meant that I had to give up certainty (as if black-and-white thinking worked) and predictability (as if it were possible to know what the future would bring). This meant I had to get into the risky world of the unknown, the spiritual realm, where there are no guarantees. Scary? You'd better believe it. Rewarding? I do believe it.

SEPTEMBER 1

"When we finish our amends most of us feel closer to our Higher Power than ever before."

—*The Twelve Steps and Twelve Traditions of Overeaters Anonymous*, 2nd ed., p. 67

Wreckage from my past keeps me focused on others. This provides a distraction from my side of the street and my part of the story. Focusing outward means I am still driven by guilt, resentment, or shame. None of these emotions permit me to be centered or to stay in the moment. They distract me as much as compulsive overeating does.

When I do a Ninth Step, I am facing my relationship problems head on. I can then say I have done what I can to right whatever wrongs I caused in the past and have changed my behavior towards people in the present. By doing this, I slowly bulldoze out the debris of shame, resentment, and guilt. I then have space to let lightness in. Spirituality is the essence of lightness.

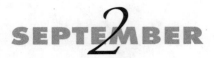

SEPTEMBER 2

"Before starting out to make amends, we must let go of any expectations of how others will receive us."

—*The Twelve Steps and Twelve Traditions of Overeaters Anonymous,* 2nd ed., p. 64

I am becoming increasingly aware of a lesson I am learning from working Step Nine. I used to feel disappointed if I didn't gain a major insight, feeling of relief, or change in my life soon after completing a Step Nine amend. Now I see that the miracle of the work is often of a different nature. Sometimes it is right in front of me, operating daily in my life. I simply do not recognize it because I am so busy searching the heavens for a blinding revelation or, at the very least, fireworks.

SEPTEMBER 3

> *"I do not need to fear failure. I need, rather, the peace of mind that comes with taking the action I have been putting off."*
>
> —*For Today*, p. 168

I had been trying to get back on track with my food for months. I kept veering off and on again, never staying long enough to get to my destination. Then I read just what I needed to help me with yet another "new beginning." This reading helps me realize that fear is a four-letter word for procrastination. How can I get away from fear? Meditation helps me recall that the answer to fear is faith. God is the engine; I am the caboose. Once again, I humbly ask for his help and guidance to kick my disease off the tracks and get my life back on the rails. I go to a meeting. I make outreach calls. I hear what I need to hear through the combined wisdom and faith of the program. I commit to follow my food plan one day at a time. I am once again clicking along the track and feeling grateful, joyful, and quite capable, thanks to God and the program.

Fear =
procrastination

SEPTEMBER 4

"Our Higher Power is the only source of help that is always available to us, always strong enough to lift us up and set our feet on the path of life."

—The Twelve Steps and Twelve Traditions of Overeaters Anonymous, 2nd ed., p. 80

Bingeing, turning to others for comfort, and addictive behaviors were my ways of coping with life before OA. Now I'm reassured by trusting that twenty-four hours a day, in every situation, God is within me to lovingly guide and direct my life. The ability to maintain abstinence through the struggle of homelessness, the pain of emotional relapse, and the fear of financial insecurity are evidence to me of a Power greater than myself.

Daily practice of prayer and meditation allows direct conscious contact with this source of healing and strength. When self-will runs riot, or character defects flare up, I trust my Higher Power to lead me back to a path of sane living. In recovery I enjoy an intimate relationship with God; spiritual friends; family; OA fellowship; and a safe, secure home. I am grateful to be beyond food obsession and harmful behaviors. A joy I could only imagine in the past is mine today, with my Higher Power guiding my life.

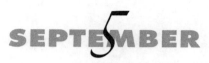
SEPTEMBER 5

"Clearly, if we were going to remain abstinent and find serenity, we had to learn better ways of dealing with other people, ways that would bring us joy instead of pain."

—*The Twelve Steps and Twelve Traditions of Overeaters Anonymous*, 2nd ed., pp. 57–58

Learning better ways of dealing with other people is a life-long process and a challenge. Yet I've learned things in OA that have helped. The first is acceptance. I had all sorts of expectations about others' abilities and behavior. I expected people to be competent, capable, and productive. I expected them to behave rationally and to be true to their word. These are my expectations for myself, and I've had to let go of them for others. I am still disappointed when someone doesn't follow through on a commitment, but I don't let it ruin my serenity.

I've also learned that I don't have to prove I'm right. I can silently agree to disagree. I put aside my pride, acknowledge another's point by saying, "You may be right," and gracefully walk away from the situation. Finally, I look for the good in people. Sometimes it requires quite a stretch, but the stretch is worth it. Focusing on the bad brings pain; the joy comes in finding the good. I'd rather have the joy!

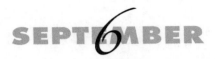

SEPTEMBER 6

"Intuition is supposed to be God's direct line into our minds and hearts."

—*The Twelve Steps and Twelve Traditions of Overeaters Anonymous,* 2nd ed., p. 20

As I repeat the Steps, they don't always look the same each time I progress through them, and yet the results are the same. My Higher Power is giving me opportunities to see the program work in my life through different situations, many of which are not the old black-and-white, "by the book" situations. Sometimes in the moment or in the not-so-distant past, I see that it was my Higher Power's presence that allowed or caused the situations to happen.

You'd think after ten years in OA, I would stop being surprised at my Higher Power's persistence and creativity. I hope that in another ten years I am still struck with awe and wonder about how my Higher Power works for, through, and in me. I hope I continue with the almost childlike innocence that my Higher Power is still with me, sometimes without my asking or approval or recognition, just as long as I am open to my intuitive sense of doing the right thing.

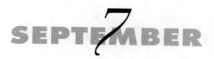
"Every character defect we have today has been useful to us at some point in our lives, and we need to recognize that fact."
—*The Twelve Steps and Twelve Traditions of Overeaters Anonymous*, 2nd ed., p. 48

After years of recovery, at times I still fear people and find it painful to tell them what I need. It's easier to stay on the road of recovery when I honor that there was a time in my life when some of the people closest to me were scary; they liked to find out what I needed, just to make sure I didn't get it. What I call a character defect today was at one time simply a survival tool. Beating myself up for using one of those old tools is as futile as bingeing: I now have two problems—the defect and the beating—instead of one. When I feel compelled to act out an old defect today, I can recognize the old hurt, put it in God's care and then act as if I possessed my defect's corresponding asset. For example, as I have wanted to please people in the past, I now seek to please my Higher Power.

8

"For many of us, our willingness to pay our own way is a sign that we are recovering and maturing emotionally."

—*The Twelve Steps and Twelve Traditions of Overeaters Anonymous*, 2nd ed., p. 134

I have learned that the Seventh Tradition is much more than putting a few dollars in the basket at a meeting. Service to my meeting, my intergroup, my region, and OA as a whole is also part of the Seventh Tradition. When I complain about something that OA is not doing, such as reaching out to newcomers, I become part of the solution when I start a newcomer's meeting. When I participate in the health of my meetings, I am taking responsibility for my part in the health of OA as a whole.

Taking responsibility is a meaningful sign of emotional and spiritual growth. It's also an opportunity to practice those spiritual Principles, since service opportunities bring out some of my character defects, such as fear, self-will run riot, or self-righteousness. I don't have to wait until I am perfect to do service, though. When those defects of character show themselves, I can work Steps Four through Nine and open myself to even more spiritual recovery.

SEPTE9MBER

"There may be times when we're faced with an important decision and want to know our Higher Power's will. Our sponsors or OA friends might suggest that we pray about it, asking God to increase our desire to take the action if we are supposed to take it, or decrease our desire if we're not supposed to take it."

—The Twelve Steps and Twelve Traditions of Overeaters Anonymous, 2nd ed., p. 80

This simple prayer has helped me in making many choices, from food selections to major life-changing decisions. Before OA, I used to rack my brain—and my nerves—over even the smallest choices because I thought I had to figure out the perfect choice that would lead to the outcomes I wanted. All that worry and stress provided a good excuse to overeat, but it never helped me make a good decision.

In Step Three, however, I turn my will and my life over to God as I understand him, and this includes my choices and their consequences. When faced with decisions today, I can take time out to ask my Higher Power's will for me, and trust that the answers will come, if I am open to listening.

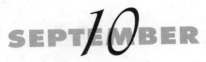

"For a compulsive overeater, eating is attached to emotions.
We are never fully satisfied, no matter how much we eat,
because we are eating for emotional reasons rather than
physical reasons."

—*A New Plan of Eating*, p. 12

Wow! This is me. This is exactly what I did. I've asked
myself how I could have weighed 214.5 pounds at 5 feet 3
inches tall. Then I read these words and found my answer.
Whenever I felt anything negative or uncomfortable, I coped
by eating. I ate when I was anxious, fearful, lonely, or tired. No
matter how much I ate, those feelings remained. Having "just
one more" never satisfied me and always hurt me. My stomach
ached from overeating.

Today, when those feelings arise, I do not eat. The
OA program has taught me to reach out for emotional
nourishment instead. I do this by calling program friends,
attending meetings, and reading the literature. The promises
are coming true, one day at a time.

SEPTEMBER 11

> "Remembering that our goal is to develop a closer conscious contact with God, prayer is simply what we do when we talk with our Higher Power, and meditation is simply a way of stilling our minds, listening, and opening our spirits to God's influence."
>
> —The Twelve Steps and Twelve Traditions of Overeaters Anonymous, 2nd ed., p. 77

I did not believe in prayer before coming to OA. For me, prayer was something that heroes and heroines practiced in order to become holy. Prayer was for the do-gooders of this world, and meditation was something for Tibetan monks. Neither practice seemed logical for ordinary people like me.

Then one day, as unexpectedly as a fresh rain shower in spring, I received a gift from the universe. I made the genuine connection between requested prayer and subsequent blessing. I finally succumbed to the idea that "nothing, absolutely nothing" is without design and purpose. It was a simple gift, really. I asked; I received. Suddenly the door of faith swung open widely enough for me to concede that God does exist, and he engineers circumstances to bring about my highest good. Thank God for OA!

SEPTEMBER 12

"There were the days when I drove my car to a junk food place.... With one hand on the steering wheel and the other fishing something out of a bag, I was lucky I never had an accident. If driving while intoxicated with food were an offense, I would have been fined countless times."

—*Lifeline Sampler*, p. 131

Many times I have recognized the insanity of my behavior. The admission that I have a problem with eating is the beginning of my willingness to recover. I am powerless over food and over my eating habits. I learn in Overeaters Anonymous that my powerlessness is the bedrock on which I can build a new life. Weakness is the glue that binds me to others in this program, and I can accept that I need help even after I have abstained from compulsive eating for years.

SEPTEMBER 13

"We pray about these things, not so we can get our way, but so we can bring our will regarding them into alignment with God's will."

—*The Twelve Steps and Twelve Traditions of Overeaters Anonymous*, 2nd ed., p. 78

So this is where I'm supposed to be. I may want something, but I no longer need to translate it into a false need. I do my best, and then I let go. If I can't be doing exactly what I want, I do what is right in front of me, accepting my Higher Power's will.

SEPTE14BER

"Many of us tried fasting, with and without a doctor's supervision. Usually we lost weight, but as soon as we started eating again, the compulsive eating behavior returned, along with the weight."

—*The Twelve Steps and Twelve Traditions of Overeaters Anonymous*, 2nd ed., p. 10

I think back to my college days when I was down to eating only one small meal a day and exercising like a maniac. I was the thinnest I have ever been. I think about the perceived power I felt, like I was winning the war with my body. But then I asked myself if I was happy. The answer surprised me. Those were some of the loneliest, unhappiest days of my life. It is very easy to forget that being thin is not the answer to my problems and starving myself is not the quick fix I want it to be. There are no quick fixes. The way to truly be a winner is by following a healthy plan of eating and working the Steps every day.

SEPTEMBER 15

"If we want to live free of the killing disease of compulsive eating, we accept help without reservation from a Power greater than ourselves."

—*The Twelve Steps and Twelve Traditions of Overeaters Anonymous,* 2nd ed., pp. 17–18

This sentence reminds me first that compulsive overeating is ultimately a killing disease. So many times I have denied its seriousness because it wasn't immediately fatal. But when I look back on the years I practiced compulsive overeating, I see how I always took the path in life that allowed me to most easily continue to practice the disease. In the meantime, the quality of my life diminished, and I gradually gave up on myself and my dreams.

Accepting help without reservation brings to mind a story about what you would do if accidentally buried alive. Immediately upon awakening, you would try to save yourself by your own devices—pushing and yelling. But then, as the compulsive overeater who hits bottom, you would reach the point of complete desperation. You would cease to care whether God was called "God," "Higher Power," or "Great Spirit." You would care only that this power was greater than yourself, and you would finally pray and accept help without reservation.

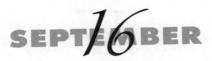

SEPTEMBER 16

"I celebrate the miracle of my new life in OA."
—*For Today*, p. 206

Little by little, the starving "hole in my soul," the open wound I carried for so long, is healing. Yesterday I was hardly hungry; coming home from work and seeing all the old familiar sights of my childhood and passing the house I grew up in did not bring me despair as it once did. It's as if a despair-proof seal is around my heart now, and only peace, serenity, and joy can seep in.

I am beginning to understand that life is just life—not a battle or contest that I must fight, rage at, and eat over. I am beginning to see my life as it is: without deception, illusion, and above all, without overeating. Denial, lies, and despair have been lifted and replaced by acceptance, truth, and joy. By accepting my past and the truth about my life today, I've found the absolute joy of realizing what a gift this life is. Now I live with an attitude of gratitude as my spiritual sight. These eyes of mine that were cloudy and dim for so long grow clearer one day at a time.

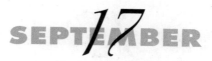
SEPTEMBER 17

> *"We believe that no amount of willpower or self-determination could have saved us. Times without number, our resolutions and plans were shattered as we saw our individual resources fail."*
>
> —*Overeaters Anonymous*, 3rd ed., p. 2

From the very beginning I was struck by the bright, often well-educated people I found in Overeaters Anonymous. I can't imagine a group who knows more about nutrition, exercise, and diets. If knowledge alone were enough to cure us, we wouldn't be here. All my knowledge did not give me the willingness I found in OA. But being willing to do something and wanting to do it are not the same. If I had waited until I wanted to abstain, I might be dead by now. Yet, I was willing to abstain, that very first day, between breakfast and lunch. I take it a day at a time, a meal at a time, with the help of my Higher Power and my OA friends.

I've learned that I can want to do something, such as eat a meal that doesn't follow my plan of eating, yet be willing not to do so. I can't do this with my own willpower. I need the program of Overeaters Anonymous, God, the Steps, and the Tools to recover, one day at a time, for the rest of my life.

SEPTEMBER 18

"What changed? My attitude! I was no longer negative, so my day was better. I felt better, had an attitude of gratitude, and started counting my blessings instead of hanging onto the negative part of my day. I felt good because I focused on my recovery instead of my disease."

—*Taste of Lifeline,* p. 77

I went to the bank, and I didn't notice friendly tellers. I didn't even appreciate that I had enough money to need a bank! I stewed over standing in line and complained if the computer was slow. At a concert I focused on rattling cough-drop wrappers or the mothball scent of the coat in the next chair. In summing up my imperfect life, I focused on "poor me" and what I was missing. No wonder I was unhappy.

What a difference OA has made. I'm learning to look for the positive in everything. A broken dryer? Thank goodness for a close laundromat. Flat tire? I'm lucky it didn't happen while I was driving. Expensive prescription? I'm grateful to live in the day of antibiotics. Now when I look up, I see that there are far more ceiling tiles that aren't stained. Thank you, Higher Power, for my new attitude of gratitude.

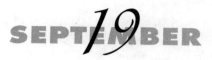

"A willingness to change is the essence of Step Six. Change is always frightening."

—*The Twelve Steps and Twelve Traditions of Overeaters Anonymous*, 2nd ed., p. 48

Growing and changing is what OA is about. Miracles and spiritual awakenings have come as a result of my slow growth. I wanted to live in the insanity of doing the same things over and over, expecting different results. It was too scary to change. Thank God I stayed around until the miracle happened. Step Six was my guide to a willingness to change. I'm grateful that I became willing to surrender to the process.

I welcome opportunities for growth and recovery—to do things differently. That is change. My program allows me to take care of myself, grow, improve, work with others, get out of myself, and make a difference in my world. I open myself each day to God's will for my life. I am willing to go to any length to keep my recovery. Each day I work the Steps and use the Tools. I live life to its fullest in recovery and refuse to give my life away to my disease. I will always be a compulsive overeater, but with my Higher Power I have the ability to change.

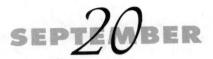

SEPTEMBER 20

"One aspect of this program that keeps us here is the promise of permanent recovery from this baffling disease."

—*The Twelve Steps and Twelve Traditions of Overeaters Anonymous*, 2nd ed., p. 69

After ten years in OA, I felt the only thing I had done right was to keep coming back. I was still overweight, obviously eating more than my body required. I knew I had changed on the inside, but, after all, I came to OA to get thin.

After a spiritual awakening while on vacation, I knew I never wanted to feel stuffed and miserable in my body again. I was finally ready to "put down the fork." At an OA retreat the following weekend, I met a lady who became my sponsor. I began a commitment to a healthy plan of eating. I achieved a normal body size and have been maintaining it for five years. I had never maintained a weight loss before. Each season, my clothes still fit—what a blessing. I am comfortable in my body. Permanent recovery is possible one day at a time. I am no longer hoping for magic. There is no magic ... but there are miracles. The promise of recovery kept me here until the miracle happened.

SEPTEMBER 21

"Our simple prayers, humbly spoken, are answered in wonderful ways as we open our lives to God's transforming power."

—*The Twelve Steps and Twelve Traditions of Overeaters Anonymous,* 2nd ed., p. 56

Humility means I recognize and accept myself as an ordinary person. Humility frees me from the bondage of self, the chain of superlatives my ego wraps around me. I no longer need to be either superstar or scum of the earth, soaring or crashing on my own merit. Instead, I can humbly ask my Higher Power to help me recognize the wisdom around me and to act on it, moment by moment, each day.

The humility I have learned in OA has given me self-esteem for the first time. I see that my intrinsic merit, like that of my fellows, was always there, whether or not I recognized it. It is a gift of the inner spirit for each of us, not a product of outside accolades for the few. Humility frees me from my comparisons and self-judgment that ultimately labeled me a loser. Humbly asking for guidance from the God of my understanding opens the door to his empowerment. I become more willing, stronger, and more confident as God's strength helps me accomplish more than I ever dreamed possible.

SEPTEMBER 22

"Although individual plans of eating are as varied as our members, … some plan—no matter how flexible or structured—is necessary."

—*The Tools of Recovery*, p. 1

How many times had I read that phrase and continued to eat without any plan? I awoke, hoped for abstinence and faced each day without a plan. No wonder I didn't lose weight. My abstinence was "three meals a day, nothing in between"—no structure, no foundation, no walls of limitation. Just eat what you want three times a day.

After six years of doing it my way, God granted me the desire for full recovery; the willingness to surrender my will, to take direction, and to follow a "plan." It's still three meals a day with nothing in between, but it now has a strong foundation based on sound nutrition, and it has walls based on quantity limits. It's not a diet, although I've given up eighty-five pounds of unnecessary weight. It's a true "plan of eating"—one that will work for the rest of my life, one day at a time.

I've just celebrated my second year of abstinence and started the maintenance of the healthy weight I now enjoy. Each time I read or hear the phrase "some plan … is necessary," I thank God for the gift of willingness he granted me two years ago.

SEPTEMBER 23

"What do we say when we talk with God? We say whatever we feel like saying."

—*The Twelve Steps and Twelve Traditions of Overeaters Anonymous*, 2nd ed., p. 77

I used to believe that the God of my understanding would not want to hear my ranting, my fears, my anger, my insecurities. Now, in recovery, I know that this God of mine is loving, understanding, and has a sense of humor. My God is always willing to love me as I am, even if I'm not. I know now what peace there is when I surrender completely and know I don't need to or want to have control. Lastly, I know that whatever form my prayers take, my Higher Power allows me to turn problems over and not eat over anything or anyone!

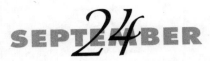

"Find a sponsor who has what you want and ask that person how they are achieving it."

—*The Tools of Recovery*, p. 2

It worked for my sponsor. Am I willing to do the same? How badly do I want to recover? I was willing to go to any lengths to practice my disease. Today, I need to do the same to achieve and maintain recovery. The Tools are there to help me. Do I use them all? I am willing to follow a plan of eating, and with God's help I can. I can go to meetings to hear how other compulsive overeaters have dealt with the challenges of life—without eating over them. I hear at meetings that eating over an issue doesn't solve the original problem. It adds a second problem as well.

My sponsor suggests that, if I am having a problem, I contact another OA member and ask, "How are you doing?" This does help me. It is not important to analyze why or how our program works. I need to take the actions that worked for my sponsor and others—and keep on coming back!

"It is only when I give up that I see the answers God puts before me. It is only when I stop trying to control that my life goes smoothly."

—*For Today*, p. 17

This is truly one of the greatest paradoxes of program. I was told early on in program that when faced with a paradox, I am looking at a profound truth. To let go is to find—to surrender is the greatest victory. My way has not worked. For my serenity I need the courage to turn it over to my Higher Power, asking for the strength to do what I cannot do myself.

The strength, the presence of my Higher Power, has always been there in my life, but my love affair with food was the block that prevented me from feeling this flow of power. The more I tried to control my food, the worse it became. By entering OA, by relinquishing my will, by asking a sponsor for help, the miracle became possible—one day at a time. Not a cure, but a daily reprieve depending on my willingness to be willing, and on my willingness to be teachable.

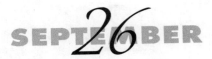

"Take the time to enjoy your meals. You deserve it."
—A Lifetime of Abstinence: One Day at a Time, p. 3

As I was growing up, meals were the time and place for verbal abuse and general arguments around the table. I remember eating while feeling a lump in my throat, choking down tears while eating as fast as I could to be sure to get enough. Enjoying, or feeling I deserved either the food or the enjoyment, were foreign to me. In program I have realized that I always felt guilt and shame as part of my reactions to a meal. Only through working the Steps have I been able to acknowledge these feelings and recognize their proper place as relics of the past. I am grateful I'm able to enjoy guilt-free and pain-free eating.

SEPTEMBER 27

"I need to be willing to give up that which attracts me in the first place."

—*For Today,* p. 132

I realized that I had to do something about my character defects if I wanted to grow spiritually. It was not a matter of choice, even if I loved my defects and could not see how I could let them go. I decided to ask my Higher Power for the willingness, and I "acted as if" until I got the willingness. I force-fed my defects with prayer until somehow my Higher Power set me free even if it took years to accomplish. I loved my defects so much, but I knew they had to go. Amazingly, God did for me what I could not do for myself. I was to ask, using Steps Nine, Ten, Eleven, and Twelve, on a daily basis. Thank you, God.

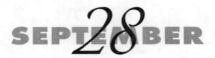

SEPTEMBER 28

"Abstinence is the beginning."
—*For Today*, p. 167

I could not work the Steps and grow spiritually without being abstinent. Putting the excess food down cleared my body and my mind so that I could be open to examine the defects of character in me that blocked me from my Higher Power. Freedom from my substance opens my mind and my heart to the changes that are necessary for me to become all that my Higher Power created me to be. When I remain in the food, the channel to my Higher Power is closed. Remaining abstinent is a priority I must have in my life if I am going to grow and change through the Twelve Steps.

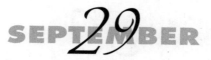

"Sought through prayer and meditation ..."
—Step Eleven

OA has taught me to PUSH (Pray Until Something Happens). Through Step Eleven, I have come to a new spiritual life. I am learning how to not just talk to God, but how to listen as well.

After I had been in OA about five years, I found myself in Italy on a bus in the rain and lost, not knowing what to do. As I sat quietly, I heard a voice within say: "Get off the bus now." Immediately I wondered what I would do if I left the bus. But since my sponsor had suggested that I always follow prompting, I got off.

As I stood there alone, lost, and afraid, I looked up and there was my hotel. I had listened and had been led to my destination. I felt such gratitude. Whenever I do follow prompting, I intuitively know how to handle the situations that used to baffle me. Prayer and meditation help me stay connected to my Higher Power, and it's that Higher Power that directs my life today.

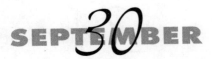

SEPTEMBER 30

"Once we compulsive eaters truly take the Third Step, we cannot fail to recover. As we live out our decision day by day, our Higher Power guides us through the remaining nine Steps."

—*The Twelve Steps and Twelve Traditions of Overeaters Anonymous*, 2nd ed., p. 23

This promise of recovery is and has been a source of comfort and confidence for me. In times of doubt or weakness, I turn to this statement and remember my commitment to recovery through the Steps. I decided to turn my will and my life over to God for safekeeping. That decision has blessed me with the ability to see the miracles that occur regularly, to avoid the extremes of my disease, and to live in balance and harmony each day of my life.

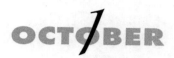

OCTOBER 1

"The purpose of Step Ten is to identify and remove from our path today's stumbling blocks."

—*The Twelve Steps and Twelve Traditions of Overeaters Anonymous,* 2nd ed., p. 70

Step Ten ever reminds me that work is to be done. While examining myself for stumbling blocks today, I find fear and anger. The fear is that nobody likes me for who I am, and the anger is because I cannot reach anyone to talk about this fear.

How can I remove these stumbling blocks so I can stop bringing pain into my life? Admitting that the fear is there is the first step toward removing it—toward relying on a Higher Power to walk me through it. I can pray for courage and make follow-up phone calls tonight to those who haven't returned mine. I can let the anger diminish. It fades now as I write about it, and always as I talk about it with a sponsor or another member.

This is an important part of my program of recovery. I need to be aware of my shortcomings and ask for their removal each day. I need to share it instead of wearing it.

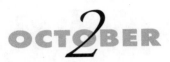

OCTOBER 2

"I cannot expect the difficulties in my life to be erased because I wish it."

—*For Today*, p. 278

We compulsive overeaters are dreamers, wishers, fantasizers. Just as I always wanted to wake up thin, get a rare wasting disease, or be a success story for a new diet drug, so did I want to wish my life problems away. Because I was heavily into food, I did not have the clarity of thought or the connection to my Higher Power or Overeaters Anonymous to help me solve problems in a reasonable way. My life was one crisis after another, one continuing drama that fueled my need for more food to reach oblivion.

How different life is since I became abstinent. Because my mind is clear and my body is strong and healthy, I can face the difficulties of life with a calmness and serenity that were totally foreign to me. I know my God walks with me, helping me over the rough spots and guiding my steps through a problem.

Today, I no longer just wish for relief from life's problems. Thanks to my Higher Power and my program, I face life's difficulties secure in the knowledge that I am carrying out God's plan for my life.

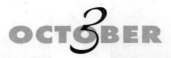

OCTOBER 3

"We had to replace our old ideas about God with a faith that works."

—*The Twelve Steps and Twelve Traditions of Overeaters Anonymous*, 2nd ed., p. 15

My old ideas of God were primarily from religious school on weekends. Although my theological education was limited, I came away with a picture of God, in the heavens, with enormous hands. He was waiting for me to sin, so he could zap me. God was there to punish, very much like a parent.

When I got involved in church choir, I began to worship God; but worship did not make a Higher Power personal to me. It was in writing and sharing with my sponsor that I became willing to see God in other ways. Those enormous hands could lift me up. They didn't need to zap me down.

A faith that works means I have to put action into my beliefs. In the morning, I ask God for guidance, but I know my Higher Power is not going to prepare breakfast, lunch, and dinner for me. I ask him for the strength and wisdom to act by making healthy food choices. God is my guide and source of hope that the obsession will be lifted each day.

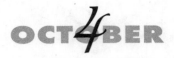

OCTOBER 4

"Our fears usually stem from our inability to trust that our basic needs will be met."

—*The Twelve Steps and Twelve Traditions of Overeaters Anonymous*, 2nd ed., p. 43

What is the worst that could happen if I trust my Higher Power to provide all that I need if I turn over my food addiction? Might I keep eating compulsively and continue on the path of self destruction? Well, that's happening now. Am I afraid that I won't find comfort and release from the stresses of life? Too much food and too much fat are the biggest stresses in my life. Relief from them would bring me comfort. Hours without compulsive thoughts about food would bring the release I seek.

I keep going to food to meet my basic needs. Food provides fuel for my body—nothing else. My need for spiritual and emotional fuel comes from within me. My Higher Power created me with all that I need. With my Higher Power's help, I will learn how to access the power within me.

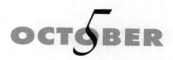

OCTOBER 5

"We now have a new reaction when we face a problem or a decision, whether it has to do with food, life, or our own runaway emotions. Instead of acting on impulse, we pause long enough to learn God's will."

—*The Twelve Steps and Twelve Traditions of Overeaters Anonymous,* 2nd ed., p. 23

I have learned to trust God to take care of me and to take charge of my compulsive eating. One day at a time he proves his strength and power and love by relieving the obsession with food. Bit by bit, I turn over my will and my life as I become conscious that I am not in a position to control a particular person, place, thing, situation, circumstance, or event. As the trust builds, I experience increasing peace of mind and a new reaction to stress, fear, anxiety, frustration, and disappointment: the desire to ask for help. Instead of the knee-jerk reaction of stuffing my face, I pray when I am in distress, either out loud or on paper to go in my God box. Peace of mind returns and the trust increases. With the trust comes another day of freedom from the insanity of compulsive eating and from the pain of living with myself.

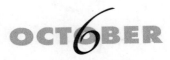

OCTOBER 6

> "We had to admit that we had not acted sanely when we responded to our children's needs for attention by yelling at them."
>
> —*The Twelve Steps and Twelve Traditions of Overeaters Anonymous*, 2nd ed., p. 11

When I first came through the doors of OA, I was a raving, raging lunatic. Sugar was my major "drug of choice," and it did really ugly things to my personality, as well as my body. When *The Twelve Steps and Twelve Traditions of Overeaters Anonymous* was published, and I read the above quote in Step Two, I was sure "you people" had been in my living room watching me. By the grace of God and OA, I've chosen not to eat sugar or eat anything compulsively since March 1990. And, on the rare occasions when I do raise my voice to my teenage son or daughter (who are both incredibly awesome people—also thanks to OA and my commitment to "keep coming back"), I almost immediately practice the Tenth Step, and we are a loving, happy family once again.

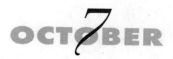

"Every character defect we have today has been useful to us at some point in our lives, and we need to recognize that fact."

—*The Twelve Steps and Twelve Traditions of Overeaters Anonymous*, 2nd ed., p. 48

As I acknowledged the usefulness of each of my character defects, I panicked. What would I become without my coping mechanisms? Surely I would flounder! Wouldn't I become an empty, dull, non-person?

Then I realized that each of my coping mechanisms has an opposite. If I am violent, then God can make me non-violent. If I am a passive person, then God can make me active. If I ask God to replace my egotism with selflessness, then I can be sure it will be done.

So when God removes my shortcomings, I will always be able to cope. After all, what better coping mechanisms are there than non-violence, action, and selflessness? Each of my character defects is replaced by its opposite, and I am equipped with a new set of survival skills—stronger, braver, and more adventurous than the old ones. God will never leave me empty. By his grace, I shall always survive.

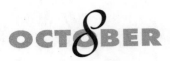

OCTOBER 8

"Humility, as we encounter it in our OA Fellowship, places us neither above nor below other people on some imagined ladder of worth."

—*The Twelve Steps and Twelve Traditions of Overeaters Anonymous*, 2nd ed., p. 52

Many of us feel discouraged in situations where our food is in order, yet the rest of our lives seem messy, out of control. We interact with people who don't think, act, or believe as we do. Some events don't follow our master plan. When we step back and realize we are trying to control other people and events, we must remember that this goes against the humility necessary for eliminating the self-righteousness and self-absorption that block our full recovery.

When we start to feel ourselves better than others, let us remember that true humility does not seek power or authority. Rather, it seeks equality and community with mankind. All we can do is live our lives, one day at a time, and trust that God has a plan. As we turn over our character defects to God in Steps Six and Seven, we humbly realize that we are not in charge; we don't know what is best for the world. As we search for the value that God has designed for each of us, we must remember that serenity and humility come with acceptance.

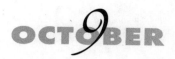

OCTOBER 9

"How does a full-grown human learn to express exuberance? Perhaps it is not possible to retrieve what was once lost, but this program of recovery comes close. The more I practice being 'as a child,' especially when I take steps three and eleven, the more my spirit is seized with an untamed joy demanding expression."

—For Today, p. 356

As an adult, I took almost everything seriously. I did not have much of a sense of humor. I neither told nor appreciated jokes. Prior to working the Twelve Step program of recovery in Overeaters Anonymous, I was terminally serious. That can really beat one down with depression, sadness, frustration, and selfishness. The Fourth through Ninth Steps led me to scoop out the garbage of my past from my spirit. Once that was gone, there was room for light—my spirit along with my Higher Power. I was able to capture the exuberance in life that was lost while I had practiced my disease of compulsive overeating. Now I am able to practice life with health. Does that mean that I am exuberant all the time? Of course not. I know I have a fatal disease; however, today I have a sense of humor, and my spirit is free to live with exuberance.

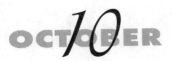

OCTOBER

"As OA members, we may serve each other by sponsoring, speaking at meetings, and doing necessary committee and other service work."

—*The Twelve Steps and Twelve Traditions of Overeaters Anonymous*, 2nd ed., p. 139

I have noticed in my home groups that people who remain in recovery are people who continue to give service. Service gives me practice at freeing myself from the bondage of self. I am gaining this freedom by concentrating on things outside myself. Every time I concentrate on what a fellow OA member is saying, I am breaking one of the strands that binds me to myself. Every time I go to a service meeting and try to speak about what is best for OA as a whole, rather than what is best for me, I am breaking one of the strands that binds me to myself. Every time I listen to a fellow compulsive overeater and encourage her recovery, I am breaking one of the strands that binds me to myself.

Every time I give service without counting the hours I give or looking for any reward, I am filled with freedom, friendship, joy, and abstinent recovery.

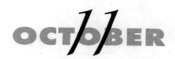

OCTOBER 11

> "Accept that we may repeatedly have the craving to eat compulsively. Experience shows us that such feelings will pass. Remember that every time we face a situation without eating compulsively it will be easier for us to abstain the next time. We can live life without compulsive eating."
>
> —Think First...

My compulsion is lifted most of the time, and I don't think about food. Sometimes, however, I still have food on my mind. I need to remember that I am not alone, that I am not a failure if I have food cravings.

I have proven to myself that when I abstain, it is easier the next time. I strengthen the habit of abstinence. If I eat compulsively, I strengthen my compulsion. I may not binge, but my food thoughts increase, and the problem increases.

My Higher Power gives me the choice to be able to say, "I don't want to eat that, to go down that path. I know what will happen." I have learned that I can turn aside, choose the path of abstinence, and continue on my way. The feelings pass, and often I forget the craving. Such a gift!

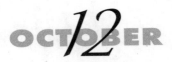

"With the compulsive overeater, not only do you get back to a normal weight, but more importantly, your life is changed, and in a sense, you're ahead of where you were before you became a compulsive overeater."

—*Overeaters Anonymous*, 3rd ed., p. 195

When I first came into OA and was failing to achieve any consistent abstinence, I kept reading this sentence. I wanted to believe it. Now I read it often to suffering newcomers. Now I can tell them from my experience that it is true. Before OA and before abstinence, I could not even imagine the potential for compassion, the potential for intelligence, the potential for spiritual life that was locked inside me by my eating. Now I know that sentence is true—I stand witness to its truth.

OCTOBER 13

> "The writing process can be very healing because, more than any other Tool of our program, it gets us in touch with our true feelings. Writing clarifies emotions."
>
> —*The Twelve Steps and Twelve Traditions of Overeaters Anonymous*, 2nd ed., pp. 60–61

Writing is the one Tool that keeps me connected with my Higher Power and lets me know when something is or is not working. It is convenient, tells no lies, and speaks clearly. I enjoy writing and find that it often benefits me more than any therapist or sponsor I have had since my OA recovery.

When I am angry, I can blow off steam. I do not have to worry if I am using "I" statements or if I am blaming someone else. When I am grateful, I can express all the wonderful things that are happening and realize it's not just because of me, but because of God and me. When something worries or distresses me, I can write and address my fears. When I am unable to make that spiritual connection, I can have a dialogue with God or the child who lives within me. I find the writing Tool indispensable to my recovery, my life, and my relationships.

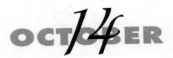

OCTOBER 14

"The only way to do meditation wrong is not to do it at all."

—*The Twelve Steps and Twelve Traditions of Overeaters Anonymous*, 2nd ed., pp. 78–79

One of the most helpful things that my sponsor taught me was this sequence for building the habit of meditating:

Develop a genuine desire to practice meditation.

Ask myself if I have meditated at the end of each day.

If I have failed to meditate, make no recriminations.

Think back through the day. Could I have done things differently?

Remind myself why I want to meditate.

Straight away, meditate.

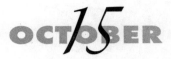

*"Our job is to be willing to let go of old attitudes that
block humility, such as low self-esteem, status seeking, and
self-righteousness."*

> —The Twelve Steps and Twelve Traditions of Overeaters
> Anonymous, 2nd ed., p. 53

When I joined OA, I heard about the necessity of being
humble. I wasn't sure exactly what members meant by
"humility," and I certainly wasn't sure I wanted any of it. But
one day I heard that to be humble meant to be "teachable."
And I thought to myself, "I think I can do that."

There were many new things for me to learn in OA: how
to look honestly at myself; how to use the Tools to work the
Twelve Steps; how to deal with old and new resentments; how
to practice the Twelve Step Principles in all my affairs. Every
day, in one way or another, I am called upon to be teachable.
For today, I am willing to give up the old ways, which did not
work, for a new way of life, which offers me recovery from my
food addiction.

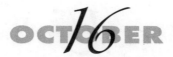

"We could 'act as if.' This didn't mean we were to be dishonestly pious or pretend we believed in God when we didn't. It meant we were free to set aside theological arguments and examine the idea of spiritual power."

—*The Twelve Steps and Twelve Traditions of Overeaters Anonymous*, 2nd ed., p. 13

This program allows me to experiment. I can test the spiritual life for myself. I do not have to accept something as true because others believe it to be true. I do not have to accept any particular description of a Higher Power before I can practice prayer and reliance on God. God as I understand him includes a God I do not understand.

I am agnostic about what God is, but I am not agnostic about the effectiveness of prayer and reliance on God. My recovery shouts beyond any doubt that prayer works, and reliance on God works.

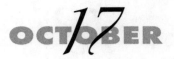

"Intuition is supposed to be God's direct line into our minds and hearts, but our problems and our self-will have interfered with this connection."

—*The Twelve Steps and Twelve Traditions of Overeaters Anonymous*, 2nd ed., p. 20

Before OA, my tendency as a compulsive overeater was to eat because I had a list of resentments, and I was going to show you. When I am overeating, overindulging in a culinary delight, or bingeing, then I am not present to win. I need to be present in my body and aware of circumstances and feelings. I am not aware of anything or anyone when I am in the food.

I have heard it said that silence is the only way we can hear God speak. To be present to hear God's message to me, I need to be willing to put away the food, the fork, the spoon, and the hand. Sometimes God speaks to me in a silent meditation, through literature, writing, or just by listening to someone at a meeting. I need to be open to receive the gift of God.

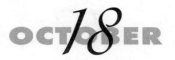

OCTOBER 18

"Once we become abstinent, the preoccupation with food diminishes and in many cases leaves us entirely."
—*Overeaters Anonymous*, 3rd ed., p. 2

What a miracle it is to be free of the obsession with food. When I first heard these words in "Our Invitation to You," they seemed like a fantasy. Now they have come true in my life.

"To eat or not to eat?" That was my question, all day long. Whether I was bingeing or restricting, food was all too often at the center of my thoughts, even if I didn't act on it.

Today, 99.9 percent of the time, I do not have any interest in eating compulsively. When the compulsion returns, I know from experience that it will pass if I do not "feed" it. Like my friends who are recovering from other addictions, I accept that to "pick up" is insanity. I am willing to wait out the discomfort, knowing it will pass, that I will have the joy of being free again and that I have been truly loving to myself. For today, I ask for the humility to go to any lengths to maintain my abstinence.

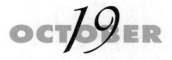

OCTOBER 19

"It is in the OA message—in our Steps and Traditions—that we find solutions to our problems. Living by these Principles has saved our lives."

— *The Twelve Steps and Twelve Traditions of Overeaters Anonymous*, 2nd ed., p. 120

The Principles of honesty, hope, faith, courage, integrity, willingness, humility, self-discipline, love, perseverance, spiritual awareness, service, unity, trust, identity, autonomy, purpose, solidarity, responsibility, fellowship, structure, neutrality, anonymity, and spirituality[3] are to be our focus. Our problems brought us to OA. OA brings us back to ourselves, to our fellow sufferers, and to God. We are more than our problems, and OA gives us a fellowship to learn this. Every day I have choices! Before OA I didn't feel I had any. All I need to do is work the program. Thank God for the people who have gone before me to help show me the way. Thank God I can now be useful to help someone else. Indeed, my life has been saved, and I am a grateful recovering compulsive overeater. What Principle will I practice today?

---

[3] The list of Principles has been updated in this edition to align with *The Twelve Steps and Twelve Traditions of Overeaters Anonymous*, 2nd ed.

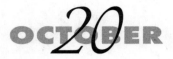

"Just as a sponsor is not responsible for the sponsee's disease, neither are we responsible for her or his recovery."

—*A Guide for Sponsors*, p. 12

As I grow in the program of Overeaters Anonymous, I need to recall how it was in the early days of abstinence. The pink cloud effect made me believe that everyone could do just as I was doing.

After having several sponsees drop out of OA, and others who found recovery in different ways, I came to the awareness that I was not "in charge." Each person has his own path. I need to follow what is best for me and let go of other people's programs.

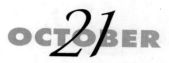

OCTOBER 21

> *"We offer our own hope, our own courage and our own experiences."*

—*Beyond Our Wildest Dreams*, p. 33

Hope was the first gift I was given. When my sponsor put her arms around my obese, smelly body, she said, "It never has to hurt like this again." In spite of my doubts, I felt hope. With that hope came courage. A deep inner courage resides within each of us. The disease has told us for so long that we don't have enough courage, but that is another of its lies. Tapping into that courage requires only the tiniest bit of willingness to change—to take a chance that the literature and people with long-term abstinence are telling the truth and that we deserve recovery.

Our experiences are our gift to the newcomer—and a reminder of how far we've come. I keep coming back because people are there for me when I need them most. It is a privilege to help keep the doors open and the lights on. Someone like I used to be is bound to walk in one day needing to hear, "It never has to hurt like this again."

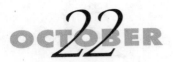
OCTOBER 22

"Nothing that happened yesterday or that may happen tomorrow is more important than NOW."

—*For Today*, p. 248

My compulsive nature wants to keep my mind occupied with events over which I have no control. I wish for some future dream and forget to work on my current defect. I want to blame the past for how I behave today. This type of thinking only causes me pain and ruins my pleasure of the present moment.

Gratefully, I now recognize this as a part of my disease, so I can turn to my Higher Power and accept events as they are, not as I might want them to be.

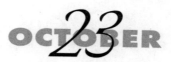

"We focused on others' faults and thought for hours about what they should do to solve their problems, while our own problems went unsolved."

—*The Twelve Steps and Twelve Traditions of Overeaters Anonymous,* 2nd ed., p. 12

I've done that for hours. I've done it for days when someone made me angry. I've done it for years when I thought about how I was brought up. When people share the mess instead of the message, at meetings or elsewhere, I realize that I am not alone in getting things backward.

I'm grateful that something (Could it be my Higher Power?) has been waking me out of these long reveries with the question, "And am I doing what I would suggest to them?" It's promising when I realize how my advice would apply to myself. It's progress when I put my advice into practice. May I tell myself early and often to mind my own business. May I take notice and act accordingly when my Higher Power gently makes a suggestion.

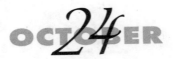

OCTOBER 24

"Gradually, we came to believe we needed to change."
—*The Twelve Steps and Twelve Traditions of Overeaters Anonymous*, 2nd ed., p. 12

Change is the key word for me in the above quote. I went into the program looking for another diet club. I kept coming back because I couldn't understand how Overeaters Anonymous worked. I kept looking and listening for the solution, and finally I found it. I would have to change the way I was eating, behaving, and thinking. The changes would happen inside myself, so the outside could change. The directions for how to change were in the Twelve Steps. Somehow, I knew that if I followed the Steps, I would achieve physical, emotional, and spiritual health. I am grateful to a program of recovery that has allowed me to understand that recovery from compulsive eating is possible if I choose to change.

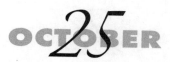

OCTOBER 25

"I didn't want the other fellows to start noticing what I ate."
—*To the Man Who Wants to Stop Compulsive Overeating, Welcome, p. 2*

We share our personal histories at meetings, as this man was doing when he told about beginning to be secretive about his eating. I'm not a man. I'm not a construction worker, as he was. No canteen truck came around onto my work site. Nothing about his story fits my life. I'm completely different from him.

Or am I? Did I really never care what people saw me eat? When did I want to hide my eating? When we talk about using the telephone as a Tool, we observe that isolation is common among us. Being secretive about eating is a symptom of our disease. What that man was sharing identified a symptom of our disease. As I further notice the quality of my behavior, I have more desire to change. Good things have happened when I've listened to others sharing in order to recognize my own symptoms. I need to notice the quality of my listening. It is a measure of my spiritual condition.

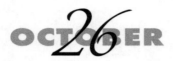

OCTOBER 26

"When has fear held me back from taking actions I might have pursued?"

—*The Twelve Steps and Twelve Traditions of Overeaters Anonymous*, 2nd ed., p. 31

I was sick with fear about my job. I was afraid I was not doing well enough. I was afraid I would be fired. If only the fear would go away, then I could get abstinent, I thought, over and over again. I was dodging the truth behind the fear. I was not doing well enough, no matter how many extra hours I worked. I had to work extra hours because I couldn't get my work done during regular work hours. The foods I craved incessantly (because I ate them) were keeping me sleepy and fogged.

I had it backwards. I had to get abstinent first, not get rid of the fear first. I'm glad those two old fellows were right, the ones who liked to say, "You can't think yourself into a new way of acting, you have to act yourself into a new way of thinking." I'm glad I accepted that I could not control my feelings, but with God-given courage I could change my actions, in spite of how I felt.

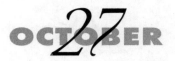

OCTOBER 27

"When I put aside what I knew ... I suddenly saw what I had missed by closing my mind."

—*For Today*, p. 89

An old Twelve Step program adage says that there are none too dumb for this program, but plenty who are too smart. For years prior to coming to OA, I was one of those "smart" ones. I knew about OA, but I still clung to the misconceptions that I could control my eating by myself; there was no God.

Since entering program, it has taken years to allow more and more of the truths of the program to permeate my defensive armor. I have had to set aside many preconceived notions, much book learning, and rationalization along the way. I now have a truly three-dimensional life as compared to the flat plane of existence I once endured without knowing any better (as bright as I was). I thank God for striking me dumb.

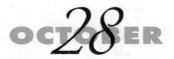

"More self-examination revealed many areas in which our lives were out of balance."

—*The Twelve Steps and Twelve Traditions of Overeaters Anonymous*, 2nd ed., p. 11

More! Can't I be done with this, at least for today? About food, I used to say, "Just one!"

What if I examine myself for just one aspect of this day that seems out of balance? Has procrastination disturbed my serenity? Has something about my use of money been undermining my calm? Has avoiding my Higher Power put a strain on me? Where has today's chief discomfort been?

It is a one-day-at-a-time program.

I ask my Higher Power to guide and strengthen me to see and to plan one action I can take towards greater serenity.

I ask my Higher Power for the power to talk about what is bothering me in the next twenty-four hours with someone in program.

What bothered me so today need not bother me so much tomorrow, because I looked honestly at myself about it, with my Higher Power, tonight.

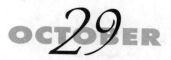
OCTOBER 29

"Most of us find that fear is at the root of many of our damaging emotions and actions."

—*The Twelve Steps and Twelve Traditions of Overeaters Anonymous*, 2nd ed., p. 43

I learned that fear hinders me—makes me pull back, keep silent, "not do" in the first place, feel left out with my friends, avoid responsibilities, and miss the moment and all it has to offer.

I have learned that once I become conscious of fear's presence, I can choose to dispel it by breathing out faith. Faith is the antidote to fear. Faith that my Higher Power is here with me, always has my best interests at heart, and will encourage and guide me to all truth, if I ask. With faith I experience this present moment and taste how good it is.

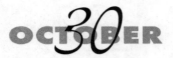
OCTOBER 30

"Were entirely ready to have God remove all these defects of character."

> —Step Six

When I was starting on Step Six, at first it seemed to me that it was unnecessary. I thought, "Why waste a whole Step on getting ready? Why not just get going on Step Seven?"

Then I remembered that when I was a child in school and we were preparing to run a foot race, the teacher would say, "Ready, set, go!" To do our best we needed to be ready. If she had just shouted, "Go!" we may not have been in our best position to start. She gave us a chance to literally put our best foot forward.

That memory made me realize the value of being ready. Now applying the same principle to Steps Six and Seven, I know I can do my best if I am entirely ready. The key to being ready is willingness, the willingness to have God remove my shortcomings.

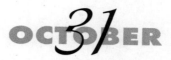

"In OA, we have discovered that humility is simply an awareness of who we really are today and a willingness to become all that we can be."

—*The Twelve Steps and Twelve Traditions of Overeaters Anonymous*, 2nd ed., p. 52

Humility is the result of knowing that I am not the doer; you are the doer, Higher Power. When I accomplish a lot, I know it is your will. When I have a bright idea, I know you are using me as a channel. When I can pray for my enemies, real or imagined, you give me the spark that makes it possible. When I continue to abstain, it is by your grace. You are my guide, my inspiration, my motivation.

NOVEMBER 1

"Sought through prayer and meditation to improve our conscious contact with God as we understood Him, praying only for knowledge of His will for us and the power to carry that out."

—Step Eleven

The hardest thing I ever had to do was let go of my self-will and turn my life over to the care of God. It has also been the best thing that has happened to me since I discovered OA.

Through my first honest prayer, I sought knowledge of God's will for me and the power to carry that out. But I didn't know how to really pray. So I started simply by talking to God. Then I would sit quietly and just let thoughts and feelings drift in and out of my mind and heart. That gave me time to hear what God might be saying back to me.

Many times when I've been sitting quietly, I have had some intuitive thoughts or ideas about how to handle a problem that is troubling me. Situations I thought were impossible have miraculously worked out because I remembered to let go of MY will and let God's will be done.

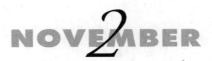

NOVEMBER 2

"We thought everything would be fine if only our bosses would recognize our worth, if only our spouses would give us the attention we needed, if only our children were well-behaved."

—*The Twelve Steps and Twelve Traditions of Overeaters Anonymous*, 2nd ed., p. 6

As the mother of two small children, I easily become trapped into thinking that my children's behavior determines my happiness. When I read this passage one evening, I realized how much this kind of thinking resembled the way I viewed food and its effects nine years ago. I used to think I would be happier if I could lose weight or stop purging. During my years in OA, I've realized that the key to my peace, not necessarily my "happiness," lies in turning my life over to my Higher Power one day at a time. When I do this, the burden of trying to "fix" the problem leaves me. My years of abstinence prove to me that my Higher Power will hold me and direct me toward action or inaction to help me do his or her will. For today, my children are in your hands, Higher Power, as is my compulsive eating. Your will, not mine, be done.

NOVEMBER 3

"We admitted we were powerless over food—that our lives had become unmanageable."

—Step One

There is a tremendous paradox between powerlessness and responsibility. When I first entered OA, an admission of powerlessness meant that there was no point in putting effort into any actions that might curtail my compulsion to overeat. It took a year's worth of experience and the patient guidance of my sponsor for me to realize that I am still responsible for doing the actions recommended by the OA program. The phrase is "powerless over food," not "powerless over footwork." Another light bulb flashed on, and so did abstinence.

NOVEMBER 4

"All of this experience, knowledge, and help is augmented by a source of wisdom inside us that becomes more powerful as we recover from compulsive eating and develop our relationship with our Higher Power through prayer and meditation."

—*The Twelve Steps and Twelve Traditions of Overeaters Anonymous*, 2nd ed., p. 20

Those of us who have trouble with the concept of God need only to look within. The solution, we learn, is always to turn from the outer to the inner. But what does this really mean? Worldly clamors will never cease. Daily, we are bombarded by false advertising, negative news, angry people, problematic schedules, glittering material goods, and enticing substances. When we pause in prayer and meditation, the answers come from seeing with our spiritual eye and listening to the voice of our soul.

Could these be visions and whisperings from God? Eventually we discover that by living abstinently, we establish or renew an acquaintance with a Higher Power who was within us all along. After all, where else would a personal God be? We learn not only to seek, but to connect with, this inner illumination and make it a working part of our lives.

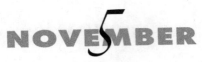

NOVEMBER 5

"Intuition is supposed to be God's direct line into our minds and hearts, but our problems and our self-will have interfered with this connection."

—*The Twelve Steps and Twelve Traditions of Overeaters Anonymous*, 2nd ed., p. 20

Food and fear blocked my connection with people and any hope for a spiritual relationship with a Higher Power. I worked hard, exercised, drank eight glasses of water, prayed, read current events, and groomed daily because I had learned that formula for living a well-rounded, fulfilling life. Every evening I could not wait to disconnect from the world and binge. When the binge began to intrude into the early afternoon, I got scared and found OA.

Following my formula for dealing with life's daily routine and challenges did not provide fulfillment. I wasted tremendous energy and thought in trying to overcome my forty-year weight problem. Seven months after I surrendered, first to a sponsor and then to a Higher Power, I lost most of my weight. My "intuition [began] to function properly, helping [me] to focus on God's will, both for [my] eating and for the living of [my life]" (*The Twelve Steps and Twelve Traditions of Overeaters Anonymous*, p. 20).

NOVEMBER 6

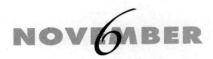

"Each group has but one primary purpose—to carry its message to the compulsive overeater who still suffers."

—Tradition Five

I love this Fellowship. I want all of us to find a lasting recovery that allows us to change. The greatest gift I can give other compulsive eaters is the same gift they have given me: proving by example that spiritual, emotional, and physical healing are truly attainable. As I find a fuller and richer recovery, I want to help others recover too.

What does it take? A simple commitment to share my recovery—not only within my group, but with sponsors and sponsees, at other meetings and beyond OA. I ask my Higher Power to help me recognize situations in which I can reach out and to guide me toward wise words and pure motivations. I commit to doing my best to strengthen the Fellowship, so it will live on for all those who keep trying to fill their souls with fast food and quick fixes.

Those who still suffer are our life blood, and we are theirs.

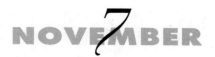

"If we could just get to the perfect weight, life would be wonderful."

—*The Twelve Steps and Twelve Traditions of Overeaters Anonymous,* 2nd ed., p. 5

I joined OA to lose weight and keep it off—something I had never managed in all my years of dieting. I believed that only my morbid obesity kept me from having a perfect life. I knew if I could "get it right," I would have no problems.

Many surprises awaited me in OA. I learned I had been using compulsive overeating to ignore deeper problems that would have overwhelmed me without the extra food. I discovered I had many more problems than I knew. OA members told me I would have to deal with my problems to get better. They said life would never be perfect—and neither would I.

These truths could have discouraged me. Instead, they freed me to be human, to make mistakes, and to try again. The glowing faces of members in recovery and their warm encouragement gave me hope that I, too, could recover if I worked the Twelve Steps. I am now recovering. My wonderful new life is better than all my fantasies of perfection.

NOVEMBER 8

"Remembering that our goal is to develop a closer conscious contact with God, prayer is simply what we do when we talk with our Higher Power, and meditation is simply a way of stilling our minds, listening, and opening our spirits to God's influence."

—*The Twelve Steps and Twelve Traditions of Overeaters Anonymous*, 2nd ed., p. 77

I always believed in God; however, Steps Three and Eleven showed me a healthy, close contact with this God. I begin every day with prayer, quiet time, and meditation. This seems to help center and calm me so I can go about my day. When I take the time each day to make contact with God, the day goes so much better. I can handle the joys and the pains without looking for and using food. At first it was easier to pray than to meditate. My magical mind was always moving, and it took a while to slow it down and to empty it, so I could listen to God speaking to me. God speaks to me in nature, in my OA friends, at meetings, and through the work of the Twelve Steps. He speaks in many ways. I just needed to learn to listen and to follow my heart, not my head. My head can lead me astray. My heart is never wrong.

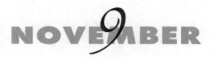

NOVEMBER 9

"Admitting the exact nature of our wrongs to another person can be a frightening prospect."

—*The Twelve Steps and Twelve Traditions of Overeaters Anonymous*, 2nd ed., p. 41

Fear that people would know the real me kept me from divulging the real me. Why risk rejection? The irony is that, in wanting to avoid rejection, I isolated myself, which put me in the same solitary, lonely position that rejection from other people would cause. But I guess it's always different if I choose it for myself. I told myself it hurt less this way, by isolating, than by having people reject me. Then came my first Fifth Step experience, and innumerable others since then, when I allowed people to know the real me, and they did not reject me. So I had been living in my self-imposed isolation all along when, in reality, people would not have isolated me. This is one more example of my tendency to do more harm to myself than other people would do to me. And it's a perfect example of the way this loving program releases me from self-defeating behavior.

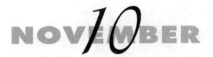

"We now needed a more reliable way of relating to a Higher Power. At this point, we learned we could 'act as if.'"

—*The Twelve Steps and Twelve Traditions of Overeaters Anonymous*, 2nd ed., p. 13

Coming into OA as an agnostic, I found that "acting as if" opened the door for me. Because my sense of separation from God and others was so persistent, I couldn't use the group as my Higher Power. I was told that experience is the best way to develop a relationship with a Higher Power. My sponsor told me to pray for help whenever I wanted to eat over something, whenever I struggled to sit with feelings or tried to work the Steps.

I set out to follow my sponsor's instructions with defiance, deciding to "act as if" just to prove it didn't work. To my amazement, it did! Over time, I have realized that it is not my job to fully define and understand this Power greater than myself. I only need to do my part—to keep an open mind spiritually, to earnestly pray for help and guidance when I need it, and to pray with gratitude for what I have received.

NOVEMBER 11

> "If we are to experience permanent recovery from compulsive overeating, we will have to repeat, day after day, the actions that have already brought us so much healing."
>
> —*The Twelve Steps and Twelve Traditions of Overeaters Anonymous*, 2nd ed., p. 69

Every time I read this passage, it brings me up short and causes me to reflect on my program. What did I do fifteen years ago to lose seventy-five pounds? What did I do over the years to arrive at the level of serenity I have now? What did I do that resulted in my Higher Power being my best friend and confidante? The really big question is, "Am I still doing the program activities today that I did in the first bloom of program?" Most of the time, I can continue to live the Principles of the Steps and use the Tools daily; I do these things more automatically and enthusiastically than ever. Time has increased my passion and commitment to our program.

When my answer to the big question is a "maybe" or a "no," I need to make adjustments in my life that give me the time and opportunity to practice program activities on a daily basis. My belief that compulsive eating is a chronic, incurable, potentially fatal disease confirms the need to persevere in the treatment plan that has worked so well for me for over fifteen years.

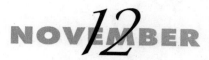

NOVEMBER 12

"Then we acted as if God were really exactly what we wanted and needed our Higher Power to be."

—*The Twelve Steps and Twelve Traditions of Overeaters Anonymous*, 2nd ed., pp. 14–15

The beginning of my recovery was the concept of God being on my side—that I wasn't left with only my own resources in this world. As I pondered the word "spiritual," I realized that it implied a vertical relationship between my God and myself, rather than a horizontal relationship that included religion and everyone else. From this standpoint, I slowly began a trusting relationship with God, finding that I could always rely on him and accepting that I could not rely on others or myself in the same way. In the twenty years since, I have had a life far better than I could ever have contemplated. God and I have shared many heartaches, but we've seen them through as only true partners can.

NOVEMBER 13

> "Many of us had asked God to help us control our weight, and this prayer hadn't worked."
>
> —*The Twelve Steps and Twelve Traditions of Overeaters Anonymous*, 2nd ed., p. 14

I have spent years praying for help with my diets and my compulsive eating. I was desperate: life felt futile because the prayers did not work. Each day I bargained with God for a reprieve. Yet I always weakened in the face of some food I loved. When I went to a Twelve Step and Twelve Tradition study meeting, however, I began to hear the solution to my problem.

Today I pray, but I ask for daily guidance instead of help with my weight. I do ask my Higher Power for help to get me through tempting situations. This lifts me to an awareness of God and changes my focus. I've prayed healing prayers for people who are ill, and I've prayed for guidance in being able to grocery shop without buying the wrong items. My weight loss results from actions I am willing to take, not from asking God to remove my fat or help me lose weight. Today I am a work in progress.

"We discover that we can learn from and work in harmony with people whose personalities we dislike, as long as we focus on OA Principles."

—*The Twelve Steps and Twelve Traditions of Overeaters Anonymous*, 2nd ed., p. 166

Tradition Twelve says that "anonymity is the spiritual foundation of all our Traditions, ever reminding us to place principles before personalities." But just what are those principles that we ought to be placing before personalities? A quick read of the Twelve Steps reveals that honesty, hope, faith, courage, integrity, willingness, humility, self-discipline, love, perseverance, spiritual awareness, and service are among them. When placing just one of these Principles before a challenging personality or situation, I reach a state of humility and thereby become "teachable." Bill W. wrote, "We alcoholics see that we must work together and hang together, else most of us will finally die alone."[4] These Principles, when applied, can help us fulfill AA's legacy and ensure that OA will be here for the next newcomer who stumbles through our door.

---

[4] *Alcoholics Anonymous*, 4th ed., p. 561

NOVEMBER 15

> *"The Eleventh Tradition is based on faith in our program and in that Power greater than ourselves that guides compulsive eaters to our doors."*
>
> —The Twelve Steps and Twelve Traditions of Overeaters Anonymous, 2nd ed., p. 161

When I am shopping, I notice obese bodies that I think would benefit from what OA has to offer. I would like to go up to them and plant the seed. However, I put myself in the other person's place and wonder how I would have felt if a stranger had approached me before I was ready.

The best way I know to plant a seed is to be the best example I can be of how OA recovery is working in my life and trust that God will provide the opportunity for me to share. I also realize that I could only try to carry the message, not that I could be successful every time. Some seeds take longer to sprout than others. If it is meant to be, it will happen in God's time.

"Going to any length means taking twelve specific steps, one day at a time, and never being finished. In the process, sanity will be restored and abstinence will become a reality."

—For Today, p. 333

A speaker at an OA convention once shared that he would have been willing to sit naked on a fireplug and hand out leaflets if that was what his recovery required. Fortunately, our program requires no single act of daring. Instead, we are shown a path to follow the rest of our lives. For those of us who sought a magic pill or diet to cure our overeating, the "fireplug program" might seem easier than practicing the Principles embodied in the Twelve Steps. Our program tells us that through "the process" of working the Steps daily, sanity and abstinence will be found. We who have followed that process for a time, and then became distracted from it, have found that sanity and abstinence are hard to maintain without it.

This program promises real and amazing recovery. Hopeless bingeing is replaced by healthy eating. Excess weight disappears without diets, purging, or excessive exercise. We can live free of the obsession with food and eating, day after day, for years at a time. But none of this is automatic. We have to be willing to live the Twelve Steps daily, in order to keep our recovery. That's what we mean by "going to any length."

NOV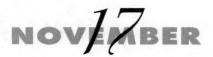EMBER

"Humility … places us neither above nor below other people on some imagined ladder of worth. It places us … on an equal footing with our fellow beings and in harmony with God."

— *The Twelve Steps and Twelve Traditions of Overeaters Anonymous*, 2nd ed., p. 52

On my bed sits a cuddly little bear I've named "Be." His kind eyes smile at me from beneath soft, brown fur, and his outstretched arms beckon me into his loving presence. He is a constant reminder of humility, of God, and of feeling "a part of."

Before I found OA, I knew well the humiliation surrounding food obsession and overeating. Today, I know something better—humility. Humility is harmony with God and acceptance of who I am at this moment.

When my self-image is low and I'm feeling depressed or "less than," I separate myself from my Higher Power. In the same way, when my self-image is grandiose, prideful, or "better than," I place distance between God and myself.

God exists in the vast, colorful space between the black-and-white extremes of depression and pride. In the middle, with God, I am free to be the authentic me and feel "a part of."

I clutch my cuddly little bear to my heart and whisper his name, "Be." He symbolizes true humility and God's presence, reminding me to just BE.

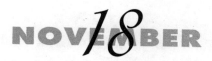
"Overeaters Anonymous believes ... compulsive eaters ...
suffer from ... a physical, emotional, and spiritual disease."

> —*When Should I Refer Someone to Overeaters*
> *Anonymous?*, p. 1

Once I got this through my head, I began to recover. When I came through the doors of Overeaters Anonymous and started to calm down, my sponsor told me that my recovery was like a three-legged stool. If the stool was to stand properly, all of its legs had to be even. The three legs of the stool represent physical recovery, emotional recovery, and spiritual recovery. Unless all the legs were even, I wouldn't—and couldn't— recover. For many years my stool had one short leg: spiritual. But now, thanks to God and this program, those legs are even. I am happy, joyous, and free.

NOVEMBER 19

> "With humble acceptance we can quietly say to our Higher Power, 'I am this way, and only with your help can I change.'"
>
> —*The Twelve Steps and Twelve Traditions of Overeaters Anonymous*, 2nd ed., p. 53

When I read this passage, I sigh. It is such a relief to be told that I can't produce the change on my own. I'm not responsible for removing the defect. The frustration of trying to do it myself, failing, and then running amok with thoughts that I am morally deficient and bad has been removed. I am given permission to turn the problem over and go on with my day. It brings me back to the present and enables me to focus on the next "right" action.

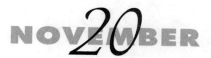

"In OA we have no program of diets and exercise, no scales, no magic pills. What we do have to offer is far greater than any of these things—a Fellowship in which we find and share the healing power of love."

> —The Twelve Steps and Twelve Traditions of Overeaters Anonymous, 2nd ed., p. 1

What, or who, is the "Power greater than ourselves" that "could restore us to sanity"? If it is simply God, why haven't we been able to pray and have our compulsion to overeat removed, our sanity restored? Why is it necessary to attend OA? Surely part of that answer is in the word "Fellowship." In the OA Fellowship, face-to-face with others who have shared our suffering, we find the power we need to recover. OA is where other people love us until we learn to love ourselves. OA is where we are buoyed by the shared experience, strength, and hope of other compulsive eaters. OA is where we can give this supportive love to others who suffer from this disease. Such giving is essential to our own recovery. Solitary reflection, prayer, meditation, reliance on God … all of these are vital to us. But so is the OA Fellowship, where we find "God with skin on" at every meeting.

NOVEMBER 21

"What we needed now was a way of remaining abstinent and living sanely through good times and bad."

—*The Twelve Steps and Twelve Traditions of Overeaters Anonymous*, 2nd ed., p. 19

When I arrived at the doors of OA, food was my master. In order to be released from its grip, I committed my food to a sponsor daily and abstained from specific foods, eating behaviors, situations, and people who were known triggers. I also attended numerous meetings. Although necessary, these actions put me at the opposite end of the food obsession.

If abstinence is to bring about a sane and useful way of life, I must have a plan that I can live with forever. The plan must be flexible when the situation warrants, allowing me to commit my food or not, to go places I had avoided, and to eat some foods I had relinquished. Once abstinence has become a habit, these things are all possible. If I find myself on unsteady ground, I must once again take the actions that worked in the beginning. Today, by God's grace, I have balance in my life and live in peaceful coexistence with food.

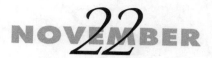

NOVEMBER 22

"... *assume a physical posture of humility as we pray.*"
—*The Twelve Steps and Twelve Traditions of Overeaters Anonymous*, 2nd ed., p. 54

I used to want things to be clearly black or white, so the rules were known and static. That way when I emerged from a time lost to bingeing, nothing would have changed. I don't want that anymore. That is stagnation and a slow, agonizing death at the hands of my disease of compulsive overeating.

Today I know that change is constant. I can choose to judge that as a negative, victimizing problem, or as a dynamic evolution toward a healthy, happy, and hopeful reality filled with wonder and awe. I choose the wonder and awe when I "assume a posture of humility," give thanks for my life to my Higher Power, and ask for another day of abstinence and the opportunity to do service for others.

"Service is its own reward."

—*The Twelve Steps and Twelve Traditions of Overeaters Anonymous*, 2nd ed., p. 142

When I came into OA, I thought that service-givers were an elite class of people, and I had to earn my place among them. I also thought service was about giving. Our Tools tell us to "give back what we have so generously been given."[5] I've discovered that service is for everyone, and everyone has something to contribute. Those who give service stay in OA longer than those who don't, and relative newcomers who take on even a small service come back to meetings. My experience tells me that when I give service, I receive more than I could ever give. When I share my experience, strength, and hope with someone, I often say just what I needed to hear.

I have learned skills I would not have today if I had not given service above the group level. I learned to work in a team and to look for what is best for the whole. I learned to speak in front of people and found that I was good at it. I learned to give workshops and facilitate meetings. Through these new skills, I embarked on a new career. Service has taught me more and given me more than I could ever have given.

---

[5] *The Tools of Recovery*, p. 6

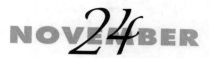
> "We have found freedom from guilt, remorse, and self-condemnation about the food we eat. We have freedom from the power food once had over us, and we have the ability to make healthy food choices."
>
> —*A Lifetime of Abstinence: One Day at a Time,* p. 6

When the mental obsession and cravings hit, I have many thoughts and actions that help me avoid that first compulsive bite. I remember the Tools and the guilt and remorse I feel after a slip or a binge. Why compound the uncomfortable feelings of food thoughts and cravings with remorse, guilt, and self-condemnation? Why not live through the food thoughts and relish the knowledge that this too shall pass if I'm willing to turn my attention to prayer, phone calls, OA service, literature, housework, or anything else until it's time for my next abstinent meal?

Often I tally the number of obsessive food thoughts I overcome during the day with my Higher Power's help. It's amazing how many times I've received the miracle of recovery in just one day! Try it; you'll like it.

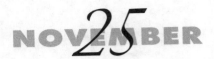

"Working the Steps will help us to let go of fear and indecision. If we are sincere, our Higher Power will give us the knowledge of our best course in life, along with the willingness and ability to follow that course, even when it seems difficult and uncomfortable."

—The Twelve Steps and Twelve Traditions of Overeaters Anonymous, 2nd ed., p. 22

My recovery depends on releasing fear and trusting God. Intellect and self-will demand attention if I let them. I feel incredible serenity when I turn to God instead. Decisions are made. Clarity and wisdom flow through me. These things only happen as I practice Steps Three and Eleven in my life. Only then can I keep my precious abstinence.

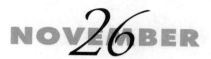

"In light of the Seventh Tradition, we begin to see more clearly what our boundaries need to be. We begin to share our vulnerability with others in OA without expecting them to shoulder our responsibilities."

—*The Twelve Steps and Twelve Traditions of Overeaters Anonymous*, 2nd ed., p. 136

Tradition Seven seems obvious at first glance: the group will pay its own way in terms of finances and service. However, a closer look reveals a more personal aspect to Tradition Seven. This Tradition shows me how to "pay" my own way in my personal life. Specifically, this means that I can't expect others to carry my burdens, perform my responsibilities, or take credit for my failures or successes. Nor am I to do those things for others. What a freeing idea this has been!

Tradition Seven seems to parallel Step Seven. Humility is the common factor. In Step Seven, we ask, in full knowledge of who we are in the sight of our Higher Power, that our shortcomings be removed; in Tradition Seven, true humility motivates us to take responsibility for ourselves in our personal lives and in the Fellowship. Once more I marvel at the wisdom and the intricacy of the Twelve Step way of life.

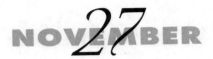

NOVEMBER 27

"The celebrations of this day will be over at midnight, and tomorrow I will wake up glad to be alive and abstinent."

—For Today, p. 151

A holiday, a birthday, a wedding: these events roll around and allow me to reach for the Tools the program has lovingly handed me.

I start my day asking the God of my understanding for help. I've learned to pick up the phone, and kind words receive me on the other end. They gently remind me of the pain I thought would grip me forever and of the most important thing I will do today: keep my abstinence.

Gratefulness envelops me, I say a quiet thank-you, and go through my day.

When I lay my head down, gratitude lulls me to sleep.

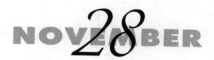

NOVEMBER 28

"Ours is a spiritual program, not a religious one."
—*The Twelve Steps and Twelve Traditions of Overeaters Anonymous*, 2nd ed., p. 12

I was raised in a religious home. I went to church every Sunday and taught Sunday school for fifteen years. However, it took OA to show me what spirituality was. Today I work several jobs and am very busy. Yet I take one hour of quiet time every morning to talk to God and pray. Before OA, I would never pray for myself, but I cannot be abstinent without God removing the obsession daily. The secret is that he wants me to ask. If I am too busy to pray, I'm busier than God intended me to be. When fear enters in, I remind myself that God did not give me the spirit of fear. In my quiet time I hear, "Fear not!" In the quietness of my mind, God gives me courage and peace.

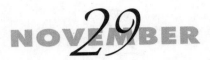

NOVEMBER 29

"Immature love tries to possess and control."
—*Overeaters Anonymous*, 3rd ed., p. 206

How many times have I become a controlling person? My life revolved around demanding that everyone do things my way and becoming obsessed with the "right" way. Then when that didn't work, I would become so submissive that others could easily victimize me. I was led into many intolerable events just to please someone else.

This program of recovery helps me to discover myself. As I have learned my own real needs, I have been able to enter into true, sharing relationships. By developing a mature love with my Higher Power and becoming a friend to myself, I can distinguish the boundaries between my will and God's will. Now choices are more blended into the question of "How important is it to my recovery?" The action of the program Principles keeps me focused on what is vital for each moment.

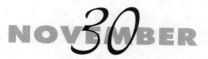

"Through prayer and meditation, we align ourselves with a Higher spiritual Power that gives us everything we need to live to our fullest potential."

—*The Twelve Steps and Twelve Traditions of Overeaters Anonymous*, 2nd ed., p. 80

I rise in the "forelight," before dawn, to align myself with the power behind the rising sun. Through a combination of prayer, meditation, reading, and writing, I put people, places, and things on the horizon. Then I sit quietly, absorbing the procession of colors from dark to dawn as the light feeds my soul and soothes my emotions. I marvel as the day offers greater fulfillment of potential in every area of my life. Simple prayers of "Thy will be done" and "Thank you, God" help me maintain my morning mood all day and night. Such spiritual food I have only discovered through continuous abstinence from compulsive overeating. My greatest potential goes beyond my own life; it exists in service to others.

DECE/MBER

"Having had a spiritual awakening as the result of these Steps, we tried to carry this message to compulsive overeaters and to practice these principles in all our affairs."

—Step Twelve

A longtimer once asked me to listen carefully to people reading Step Twelve and see how many people read "as a result of these Steps," instead of "as the result of these Steps." Sure enough, I heard it a number of times. The person explained that the Steps were worded so specifically so that the meaning would be absolutely clear. After working through all Twelve Steps, my result would be to have a spiritual awakening. It would not be one of a number of results, it would be THE result. This clarifies what I am working toward when I go through the Steps to the best of my ability. I am trying to have a spiritual awakening that will allow me to stop eating compulsively, certainly the result I want from working the OA program. From that, everything I need in life will follow.

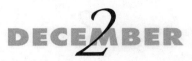

DECEMBER 2

"I can hold onto fear that serves the purpose of keeping compulsion alive, or I can turn my life—one moment at a time—over to my Higher Power."

—*For Today*, p. 104

Fear and anxiety have haunted my entire life. They have also been a constant challenge in my recovery from compulsive overeating. Forming a relationship with a Higher Power, whom I call God, has resulted in several years of abstinence and an ability to walk through fearful situations. In order to grow emotionally and spiritually, I need to take risks; that brings up fear. But I have learned that it does not matter how afraid I am. I can show up anyway. I pray and ask God to help me, and I've never been disappointed. Each time I conquer something that I am afraid to do, it boosts my self-esteem and enables me to take the next risk. The combination of abstinence and a reliance on God has given me courage. I will never be without fear, but with God's help, I have been able to face my fears abstinently and accomplish things I never thought possible.

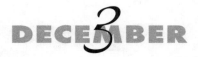

DECEMBER 3

"Pray to God, but continue to row to shore."

—Russian proverb as quoted in *For Today*, p. 136

Surrender does not mean that I take no action; it means that I take action and surrender the results. I have learned that my imagination is limited. I am lucky to see two options, though there may be dozens. If I do what is suggested and let go of the results, I often find better results than I could have imagined. In Overeaters Anonymous, I have learned that the Twelve Steps provide a way of working through a problem. This is the equivalent of "rowing to shore." First I work Steps One through Three, and then I take the action Steps, Four through Nine. This way, I can rid myself of my character defects, one at a time.

I realized this while working through the Steps for the first time. After completing Steps Six and Seven, I was relieved of anger as a driving force in my life. It was a tremendous relief and a strong incentive to work the rest of the Steps and to continue working them to this day. The image of me rowing a boat is a good one. I don't have to be at the mercy of the currents, nor do I need to attempt to control nature. I can do the best I can, knowing that is enough.

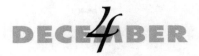

DECEMBER 4

> *"Step Eleven encourages us to practice prayer, to continue talking to our Higher Power daily, even when it seems like a senseless exercise."*
>
> —The Twelve Steps and Twelve Traditions of Overeaters Anonymous, 2nd ed., p. 76

Prayer changes things. I am very clear about that. In my former life as a desperate, insane food addict, I used my brain well, but I was a spiritual agnostic. I just didn't believe in anything. And then, at my sponsor's suggestion, I started saying "good morning" to God every day, just to see what happened. The result was extraordinary. God came toward me when I came toward God. He took hold of my empty soul and filled it with his presence.

Talking to God every day is now part of my life—I simply can't live without it. I see prayer as an exercise of the soul, just as though it is an exercise of the brain. I have to deal with my life now through both my brain and my soul. And just as no thought is ever useless or wasted, neither is a single prayer. Prayer changes things. And when I don't like the changes, I can at least be sure that they have come from God.

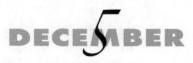

DECEMBER 5

"I am thankful that the pain of compulsive overeating gave me the vision not to try to change the world or other people or situations or even myself, but to do the footwork and leave change up to my Higher Power."

—*For Today*, p. 121

During the black, bleak time before I found abstinence and the Steps, I was filled with fear, depression, loneliness, despair, and self-pity. I was always looking for something to "fix" me: a relationship, more money, the perfect diet, a better shrink. Mostly I wanted someone to take care of me forever. Guess what? That's exactly what I've found in recovery—a Higher Power who takes care of me forever. I no longer doubt that there is such a Power. There's too much proof that something responds to me when I'm willing to change. My only job is to do the footwork and to trust. I believe this search for connection to a Higher Power is the "hole" I tried to fill with food. It is as if I wandered away from home long ago in an amnesia so deep, I didn't even know I was lost. But something kept calling me to a pathway of healing and hope. It called me to OA. It called me home.

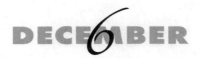
"Before we joined the OA Fellowship, our prayers for help might have gone unanswered simply because we were never meant to face this disease in isolation."

—*The Twelve Steps and Twelve Traditions of Overeaters Anonymous*, 2nd ed., p. 14

As a child, I remember praying to a God I didn't believe in. I prayed to be thin while continuing to eat whatever and whenever I wanted. Over the years, my "prayers" became pleas: if you help me stop bingeing, I will always—or never again—do ...

By the time I started going to OA meetings, at age thirty-four in 1985, I had no need for a God who didn't help me (or so I thought). In fact, I crossed out the word "God" throughout my copy of AA's Big Book. After all, I came to OA to lose weight. I had no idea that physical recovery needed the accompaniment of spiritual and emotional growth.

The OA *Twelve and Twelve* explained it differently: I wasn't meant to recover alone. I needed the OA Fellowship, a Power greater than myself, to help me. So, in fact my prayers had been answered. I later heard it said that our prayers are always answered positively: either "Yes, but not now," or "I have something better in mind."

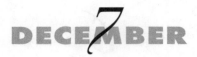

DECEMBER 7

"We're always happy to share our secret: the Twelve Steps of Overeaters Anonymous, which empower each of us to live well and be well, one day at a time."

— *The Twelve Steps and Twelve Traditions of Overeaters Anonymous*, 2nd ed., p. 87

Over the years that each of us have spent or will spend on our individual recoveries, we develop certain ideas and philosophies that help us walk the magnificent journey of physical, emotional, and spiritual discovery. One of mine is a belief in the Five "Ps" of Program: practice, prayer, perseverance, patience, and progress. If I want to stay in recovery on all three levels, I need to do these things every day. I practice the program to the best of my ability; no half measures will do. Half measures get half results, and I'm not satisfied with that anymore. I expand my spiritual awareness through prayer. I pray to the God of my understanding that I may know his will for me, and I pray for the willingness and power to carry that out. Spiritual awareness is my breath of life, and it takes perseverance to sustain that life. I learn patience by waiting for the fruits of my efforts, knowing they will come in time.

You will be amazed and grateful for the progress you make. Your spirit will soar, and you will be able to show your gratitude by passing on the secret of your recovery—the Twelve Steps—to others.

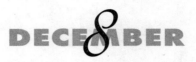

DECEMBER 8

"The only requirement for OA membership is a desire to stop eating compulsively."

—Tradition Three

I get so much comfort from this. I have the desire because I showed up at that very first meeting. I have kept coming back, abstinent or in relapse, because OA is the only thing that has worked for me. I have a "living" problem, and no diet has ever taught me how to cope with life. Food, people, or material things can always fail me. The only real thing I can count on is my Higher Power to see me through whatever today may bring.

Some days I have to act as if. I must act as if I have the desire to not eat compulsively and act as if I believe that my Higher Power is there for me. If I take this action, my Higher Power takes care of my needs; the obsession is lifted, and abstinence comes. So for today, I will not give up. I will just keep trying, with my Higher Power helping me along the way. I will become a much happier person with my life held in my Higher Power's loving embrace.

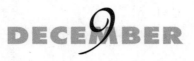

"Many of us begin and end our day with prayer and meditation."

—The Twelve Steps and Twelve Traditions of Overeaters
Anonymous, 2nd ed., p. 76

The time between sleeping and waking is when I stir up the thoughts in which I'll marinate all day. Those thoughts easily revolve around who's done me wrong and why I'm so helpless against their conniving ways. By working the Eleventh Step as soon as I am conscious each day, I become powerless—rather than helpless.

Upon awakening, I ask my Higher Power to divorce my thoughts from self-pity, dishonesty, and self-seeking. When I ask for help with my motives, I receive peaceful clarity in my thinking process. The clarity gives me more mental energy for problem-solving. It releases me from the sludge of judging other people and helps me listen to God's will. Today, this healthy spiritual condition allows me to react sanely and normally to food.

"As we repeatedly act on Step Ten, we begin to see the remarkable way the Steps can, from now on, continue to remove unnecessary turmoil and pain from our lives.... More gifts are in store for us as we continue working the program and experiencing the miracle of permanent recovery, one day at a time."

—The Twelve Steps and Twelve Traditions of Overeaters Anonymous, 2nd ed., p. 74

Ours is a disease of the attitudes. However, the years I've spent in OA have shown me that although my disease is progressive, so is my recovery. When I was active in my eating disorder, I hated everything about my life. My world consisted of binges, blame, fear, shame, jealousy, and rage. I was imprisoned by unrealistic expectations of people, bitterly resenting their imperfections. I also hated myself because I couldn't stop eating. Negativity breeds hopelessness, and I was trapped.

Recovery teaches me that my gratitude and serenity snowball, just like my negative attitudes did. As I work the Twelve Steps of this program, it becomes fulfilling to focus on the good in my life. It doesn't always come easily; sometimes I struggle to think positively. But when my attitudes slip, I know there's hope. Now my world consists of daily miracles, both large and small, that keep the light in my eyes and lightness in my heart. Positive thinking breeds acceptance, and today I am free.

DECEMBER 11

"Recovery is a journey, and the Twelve Step program is the road we travel together in OA."

—*The Twelve Steps and Twelve Traditions of Overeaters Anonymous*, 2nd ed., p. 108

I have grown to understand that my commitment to OA recovery is a commitment to travel a specific road, a commitment to take a journey. To start this journey, I did not need to envision any end of the journey. I only needed to know that where I was had become intolerable. In fact, the Steps have taken me to a place I could not have imagined before I started. Looking back, I am filled with gratitude. Looking forward, I see only mists and cannot make out where the road leads. This road leads to something beyond my understanding. Yet I am not afraid of what the mists hide. I have learned from experience that the most joyous thing in my life is my commitment to the OA journey of recovery.

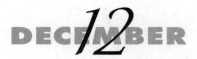

DECEMBER 12

"The Twelfth Step invites us to continue the journey one day at a time for the rest of our lives. We need to keep moving forward in recovery, keep developing our spiritual consciousness, if we are to remain spiritually awake and fully alive."

—The Twelve Steps and Twelve Traditions of Overeaters Anonymous, 2nd ed., p. 82

There is one fear that I hope my Higher Power never relieves me of: the fear of complacency. Several times I've come into this program full of pain and despair. And then later I've left cocky, convinced I was cured. Two things have led to my downfalls: the refusal to surrender to Step One and complacency.

Today I'm convinced that I'm powerless over food, and if I allow complacency in my program, my life will become unmanageable. When I don't take time to read the literature, make phone calls, provide service, or talk to my Higher Power, I have stopped moving forward in recovery. My disease has won a battle, and it doesn't take many battles for my disease to declare victory. Complacency is a powerful, frightening aspect of my disease. Each day I need to remember that this journey I'm on is full of hope and life. If I stay on its path, my Higher Power will lead me forward.

DECEMBER 13

"Those who are prone to stuff themselves with food that makes their bodies unsightly are refusing the food that satisfies and soothes the unhappy soul within."

—*Overeaters Anonymous*, 3rd ed., p. 205

My food fear has lessened since coming into program. I can walk down the binge-food aisle in the grocery store. I no longer fear going to a party because of the food that will be there. I know I can recoil from it and rest in the arms of God. I no longer feel obligated to eat someone else's gift of food. What has changed? I have given my life and my will over to the God of my understanding. My life is service. I am no longer dieting, but I don't stuff myself either. I've simply made a choice to abstain from my binge foods and work the Twelve Steps. The promises are coming true for me. God is keeping me unharmed.

"We go to meetings, we make an effort to express our feelings openly, and we act as if the power to change, to abstain from compulsive overeating is already ours."

—*For Today*, p. 8

I have always been a person who sees "the big picture" and plans ahead. At those first few meetings, I couldn't comprehend that my abstinence and recovery were not a lifetime commitment. When stumbling through the beginning of my recovery, I came upon the phrase of living and acting as if—as if I am abstinent, as if I have a solid relationship with God, as if I have a sponsor, and as if I am indeed recovering.

That simple mental adjustment has helped immeasurably. I have come from acting as if to actually being abstinent, to having a relationship with God, to living one day at a time, to having a sponsor (and now being one), and to actually recovering. Learning to live in the moment has been a blessing. I no longer fret about what hasn't been done, or what has already happened. I've learned to "just be." I can acknowledge that for today, I am abstinent and grateful. I'm no longer in the driver's seat. That simple thought could never have happened without OA.

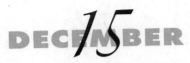

DECEMBER 15

"What do I need to write about? I do not have to be afraid to look into my heart and put down what I find."

—*For Today*, p. 178

Tonight I am withdrawing into senseless activity. Why? What are my feelings? ANGER—I fear anger because I have used it to hurt others and myself. It is safer to hide it in some activity.

Anger. Can I recognize it and deal with it without destroying others or myself? Yes, with the Twelve Steps of OA and its Tools, I can. I can write about my anger and, as I do, I discover the more basic emotions of frustration, anxiety, and loss of control.

As I write, my anger lessens. I can talk to my sponsor and other OA members who can help me understand this anger and can help me let go and turn it over to God. Since OA, I no longer have to be afraid to look at my anger and put down what I find there. Then I can deal with it constructively.

I can live honestly with myself as I recognize and write about my feelings.

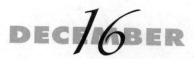
"Each twenty-four hours is vital and precious when I totally turn over my life and my will to a Power that has more wisdom than I can ever hope to have.

I don't know how I got where I am, or where I'm going; but my Higher Power does. So I'll trust God to guide me, and pray for the good sense to listen."

—*Lifeline Sampler*, p. 212

   This program is so simple. Why do I make it so difficult? I just need to ask my Higher Power to guide me through today, this one singular day. At night, I can thank my Higher Power for whatever the day has brought me, regardless of my perceptions of good or bad events. There are lessons to be learned with every experience I encounter. If I do not recognize what I have learned, I am destined to repeat the lesson. If I truly believe everything is happening for a reason, I can be grateful for whatever the day has brought me. By following this simple program every day, I will begin to receive all the gifts promised to me by the program. For today, let me remember to keep it simple.

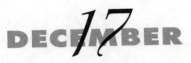

DECEMBER 17

"Those of us who live this program don't simply carry the message; we are the message."

—The Twelve Steps and Twelve Traditions of Overeaters Anonymous, 2nd ed., pp. 86–87

Like much of our literature, in simple language we are given a blueprint of how to convey the most effective message to the newcomer. It emphasizes our experience, rather than our opinions; our progress, instead of our expertise; and our trust in the future, rather than our regrets over the past. The power of the individual example is undeniably one of OA's greatest assets. Our stories are full of courage and self-sacrifice; of hard-earned triumphs and reluctant surrenders; of embarrassments and inspiring lessons in humility.

Such is the essence of our recovery. Measured in individual days, OA can offer otherwise hopeless compulsive overeaters a lifetime of opportunities to renew and rebuild, to grow and change, and to pass their experience along to the next newcomer. This process has proven to be a miracle to those of us who have given ourselves over to it completely.

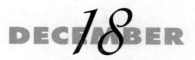

DECEMBER 18

"If we are to experience permanent recovery from compulsive overeating, we will have to repeat, day after day, the actions that have already brought us so much healing."

—The Twelve Steps and Twelve Traditions of Overeaters Anonymous, 2nd ed., p. 69

There are those gray, bleak days when I don't feel like doing what I need to do to recover. I'm tired of the effort. I want to give up, but I stop and reflect. If I quit making an effort, I'll slide backwards. And backwards, for me, means only one thing—the hell of compulsive overeating and all the accompanying mental, physical, and spiritual anguish it brings.

So I pray for the willingness to do whatever my Higher Power nudges me to do. Then I get my body in motion and do it! I may need to make amends, spend time with my children, be honest with someone, carry out a responsibility, get to a meeting, make a phone call, read, write, or give service. And then once again, I experience the healing and recovery that taking action on the Twelve Steps always brings.

DECEMBER 19

"Taking Step Three shows our willingness to live by God's will, one day at a time."

—*The Twelve Steps and Twelve Traditions of Overeaters Anonymous*, 2nd ed., p. 23

Trying to understand Step Three, I asked how to turn my will and my life over to God as I understand him. What was I supposed to do? Then I read this passage, and a thought came to me: How often are we told to work the program? God was my employer! In following the program to best of my ability, I wasn't just making phone calls, going to meetings, sponsoring, following a food plan, and using the Steps; I was doing a job. I could do this job for the rest of my life and never be fired. I could do my "recovery job" anytime, anywhere! This idea gave me tremendous comfort and a sense of usefulness and purpose. It also showed that I need to leave enough time in my life for my program, just as I would for any job. And every day that I don't eat compulsively is payday!

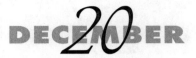

DECEMBER 20

"Have I let the needs of others govern me while I ignore my own needs?"

—The Twelve Steps and Twelve Traditions of Overeaters
Anonymous, 2nd ed., p. 32

Once I believed that I needed to allow others' expectations to influence my food choices. In OA I learned that unless force was being used, I was the one making the food decisions. I had to admit that no one had persuaded me to eat anything. I've discovered that most people are too preoccupied to notice what others eat. The few who have focused on my food choices have had their own addiction problems.

For example, one acquaintance urged me to eat foods that I had eaten in the past. I realized that she was struggling with her own lack of control. Joining her in a binge would have harmed me and would not have helped her—better to be an example of hope. Now when someone comments on my food choices, I reply that I feel better when I follow my food plan. No one has ever responded by urging me to do something that would make me feel worse.

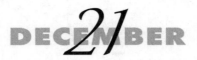

DECEMBER 21

"As OA members, we may serve each other by sponsoring, speaking at meetings, and doing necessary committee and other service work. For this, none of us receive payment in money. Our reward is something money can't buy—our own personal recovery."

—*The Twelve Steps and Twelve Traditions of Overeaters Anonymous*, 2nd ed., p. 139

I thought I would offer service to give back to OA some of what it gave to me. Was I surprised! I do contribute, and I do give back. What surprised me was that even when I am doing service, I get far more than I give. When I study the Steps with a sponsee, I inevitably learn something new, something I needed to learn. When I share my experience, I often say just what I needed to hear. When I am having a difficult time in my life, the knowledge that one day I will be able to share my experience, strength, and hope with someone who is having the same difficulty makes it easier.

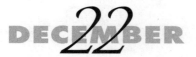

DECEMBER 22

"Denial of the truth leads to destruction."
　　—*The Twelve Steps and Twelve Traditions of Overeaters Anonymous*, 2nd ed., p. 7

When I first came to OA, admitting I was a compulsive overeater was a big step toward my recovery. What about today? Have I said the words "I am a compulsive overeater" so many times that they have lost their meaning for me? I need to keep in mind that while I've been recovering in the OA rooms, my disease has been doing push-ups out in the hall. My compulsion to overeat is cunning, baffling, powerful—and patient. If I am wanting to eat inappropriately or to overeat, it will do me no good to deny to myself what's going on or seek to hide it from others. That kind of egotistical pride will surely lead to relapse.

It doesn't matter how long I've been working the Steps or how many service positions I've held or how long I've been abstaining or how much physical recovery I have. Today, if I'm wanting to overeat, I need to call someone and talk about it. I need to say those humble, magic words I said when I first came to OA: "I need help." In this way, I admit to God, to myself, and to another human being the exact nature of what's wrong with me today. When I stop denying the truth, it loses its power to destroy me.

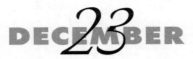

DECEMBER 23

"When we keep OA's Eighth Tradition, we discover a beautiful spirit of caring service, which becomes a powerful factor in our healing."

—*The Twelve Steps and Twelve Traditions of Overeaters Anonymous*, 2nd ed., p. 143

The recovery and growth I've received from doing service astounds me. By sponsoring, I learned how to be in a relationship. By leading workshops, I learned how to be a facilitator. By chairing a committee, I learned how to work on a team and was able to transfer those skills and that knowledge to my family. I learned how to listen and how to compromise for the good of OA as a whole, and so I learned how to listen and compromise for the good of my family or my relationship. I learned that I don't have to do it all. I learned that "group conscience" works in many situations, including work and home. I learned how to speak in front of a group of people and have made that my professional career. I learned that I am intelligent and capable. I am learning who I really am and who I am becoming. All of this for the small price of some of my time and energy. The rewards have been immeasurable.

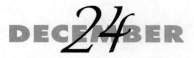
"Alas, it is not enough to want to be rid of the unpleasant side effects of my illness. I need to be willing to give up that which attracts me in the first place: the gratification, sedation or whatever other payoff I get for practicing my compulsion."

—For Today, p. 132

The main payoff I get from compulsive eating is relief from loneliness. As a small child, I sought friendship in food. For as long as I can remember, food has been a companion to console me when I had no one else to turn to, to look after me when I thought no one else cared. My loneliness has decreased since I came to OA. I feel at home here. I am one among many.

I was ready to give up being overweight, but not to give up the friendship I found in food. In OA I learned to replace food with love of myself and of others. I've let go of compulsive eating, one day at a time, for more than nine years. God has replaced food with something incomparably better: a happy, joyous life.

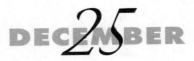

DECEMBER 25

"Thinking of compulsively eating is not compulsively eating. We do not have to act on our feelings. The worst thing we can do is try to talk ourselves out of it…. We can abstain, no matter what."

—*A New Plan of Eating*, p. 11

My sponsor says, "Stay out of your head. It's a dangerous neighborhood." A comedian once said, "Whenever I get into an argument with myself, I always lose!"

If I listen to the voices in my head, they can rationalize me into a runaway relapse. Thinking just doesn't work for me.

What works for me is to get out of my head and into my heart with heartfelt prayer and an attitude of gratitude.

What works for me is to get out of my head and into action, working the Steps, and using those wonderful Tools: a plan of eating, meetings, telephone, literature, action plan, anonymity, sponsorship, writing, and service.

I can abstain, no matter what. Thank you, OA!

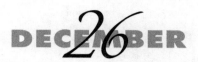

DECEMBER 26

"The powerful force that brought me to OA is ready to lead me to the promises of this program."

—*For Today*, p. 335

No human power can relieve me when I feel empty. God can and will give me peace! All I need to do is read, write, pray, stay close to my Higher Power and OA, and work the Steps. The solution is so much kinder to me than the disease ever was.

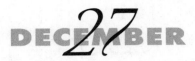

DECEMBER 27

"It is essential that all of us understand and respect anonymity if OA is to survive and we are to find recovery here."

—*The Twelve Steps and Twelve Traditions of Overeaters Anonymous*, 2nd ed., p. 164

It's not often you see the words "It is essential." This tells me how important anonymity is. OA's survival and my recovery depends on it. What does this mean? For me, it means that I always hold in confidence what I hear at a meeting or from another OA member. It means that no matter what, I maintain my anonymity at the level of press, radio, films, television and other public media of communication. For me, it also means that I let people in OA know my last name so that if I am needed, I can be found. It means that I don't place myself above or below anyone else. It reminds me that we are all equal. It tells me that my job is of no importance. What counts is that we are all compulsive overeaters trying to recover through the Twelve Steps and Twelve Traditions of Overeaters Anonymous.

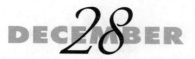

DECEMBER 28

*"'I would if I could, my friend, but—as it is for me—
the problem is within.' ...*

*I am completely honest in taking stock of myself so I can learn
why I feel as I do about myself."*

—*For Today,* p. 277

It seems that for most of my life I have been searching for
the answer book. In school, there was always one definitive
answer, and the teacher had all the answers. Unfortunately, in
life there is no one right or wrong way to do something. There
are no answer books. Yet some experts believe that their book
or product will solve whatever my current problem may be.

I finally realized that I have been searching in all the wrong
places. No one has my answers; they don't even know what
the question is. I believe that all my answers are within me.
The difficulty lies in looking within, something I'm incapable
of doing alone. I need the love, help, and support from others.
What I have been looking for is not the answer, but the
question.

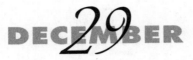

DECEMBER 29

"Sponsors, OA friends, meetings, and literature are wonderful sources of help for us. We wouldn't want to be without any of these resources because we often find God speaks to us through them."

—*The Twelve Steps and Twelve Traditions of Overeaters Anonymous*, 2nd ed., p. 80

As a compulsive overeater, I tend to overdo almost everything, including service. I think I naturally want to mother and take care of everyone, putting myself at the bottom of the list.

My sponsor recognizes my symptoms and gently reminds me that I may have too many things on my plate. She suggests that I check with my Higher Power before committing to something that may put me into overload. Sometimes she asks, "Do you need to decide today?" My response is usually "no." This means that I can let it go for a while and deal with it if it comes up again. God speaks to me through other people, especially my sponsor, when I listen.

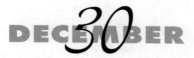

DECEMBER 30

"God grant me the serenity to accept the things I cannot change, courage to change the things I can, and wisdom to know the difference."

—Serenity Prayer

I was spending most of my energy on things I could not change, worrying, fretting, and trying to make them come out "my" way. Meanwhile, I was ignoring things that I could change, spinning my wheels where they did the least good. No wonder I felt so much stress and self-loathing.

Now, when I find myself troubled by an issue or situation, I think about it while I say the Serenity Prayer. If it is something I can change, I think of the steps I can take to begin the change, and I pray for the willingness to take action. If it is something I cannot change, I turn it over to my Higher Power and pray for the willingness to accept it. This exercise brings serenity to my life and helps me feel God's presence.

DECEMBER 31

"We are promised 'a life of sane and happy usefulness'[6] as the result of working the Twelve Steps."

—*The Tools of Recovery*, p. 6

"Who would want that?" That was my reaction to reading this line for the first time, nearly seventeen years ago. I wanted a slim body and plenty of money, not service to others. Today I am convinced that my Higher Power led me to Overeaters Anonymous. I got far more that I bargained for when I walked in the OA doors.

It had not occurred to me to try a spiritual solution to deal with what I thought was a physical problem. I had been compulsively overeating nearly all my life before coming to OA. I just didn't know there was a name for what I did. I am very grateful that I have kept coming back to meetings regularly, week after week. My Higher Power continues to challenge me to love and accept myself just as I am today and to pass on the message that recovery from this disease is possible. "Sane and happy usefulness" to myself and others is something I value and strive for today, one day at a time.

It has been a unique experience for me to reach out to still-suffering compulsive overeaters and know that there is a solution in OA, if they want it.

---

[6] *Alcoholics Anonymous*, 4th ed., p. 130

INDEX

The Twelve Steps of Overeaters Anonymous

1. We admitted we were powerless over food—that our lives had become unmanageable.

2. Came to believe that a Power greater than ourselves could restore us to sanity.

3. Made a decision to turn our will and our lives over to the care of God *as we understood Him.*

4. Made a searching and fearless moral inventory of ourselves.

5. Admitted to God, to ourselves and to another human being the exact nature of our wrongs.

6. Were entirely ready to have God remove all these defects of character.

7. Humbly asked Him to remove our shortcomings.

8. Made a list of all persons we had harmed, and became willing to make amends to them all.

9. Made direct amends to such people wherever possible, except when to do so would injure them or others.

10. Continued to take personal inventory and when we were wrong, promptly admitted it.

11. Sought through prayer and meditation to improve our conscious contact with God *as we understood Him,* praying only for knowledge of His will for us and the power to carry that out.

12. Having had a spiritual awakening as the result of these Steps, we tried to carry this message to compulsive overeaters and to practice these principles in all our affairs.

Permission to use the Twelve Steps of Alcoholics Anonymous for adaptation granted by AA World Services, Inc.

The Spiritual Principles in the Twelve Steps

Step One: Honesty

Step Two: Hope

Step Three: Faith

Step Four: Courage

Step Five: Integrity

Step Six: Willingness

Step Seven: Humility

Step Eight: Self-discipline

Step Nine: Love

Step Ten: Perseverance

Step Eleven: Spiritual Awareness

Step Twelve: Service

The Twelve Traditions of Overeaters Anonymous

1. Our common welfare should come first; personal recovery depends upon OA unity.

2. For our group purpose there is but one ultimate authority—a loving God as He may express Himself in our group conscience. Our leaders are but trusted servants; they do not govern.

3. The only requirement for OA membership is a desire to stop eating compulsively.

4. Each group should be autonomous except in matters affecting other groups or OA as a whole.

5. Each group has but one primary purpose—to carry its message to the compulsive overeater who still suffers.

6. An OA group ought never endorse, finance or lend the OA name to any related facility or outside enterprise, lest problems of money, property and prestige divert us from our primary purpose.

7. Every OA group ought to be fully self-supporting, declining outside contributions.

8. Overeaters Anonymous should remain forever non-professional, but our service centers may employ special workers.

9. OA, as such, ought never be organized; but we may create service boards or committees directly responsible to those they serve.

10. Overeaters Anonymous has no opinion on outside issues; hence, the OA name ought never be drawn into public controversy.

11. Our public relations policy is based on attraction rather than promotion; we need always maintain personal anonymity at the level of press, radio, films, television and other public media of communication.

12. Anonymity is the spiritual foundation of all these Traditions, ever reminding us to place principles before personalities.

The Spiritual Principles in the Twelve Traditions

Tradition One:	Unity
Tradition Two:	Trust
Tradition Three:	Identity
Tradition Four:	Autonomy
Tradition Five:	Purpose
Tradition Six:	Solidarity
Tradition Seven:	Responsibility
Tradition Eight:	Fellowship
Tradition Nine:	Structure
Tradition Ten:	Neutrality
Tradition Eleven:	Anonymity
Tradition Twelve:	Spirituality